Mastering Pain

Mastering Pain

A Twelve-step program for
coping with chronic pain
by DR. RICHARD A. STERNBACH

G. P. PUTNAM'S SONS / New York

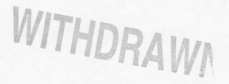

G. P. Putnam's Sons
Publishers Since 1838
200 Madison Avenue
New York, NY 10016

Library of Congress Cataloging-in-Publication Data

Sternbach, Richard A.
    Mastering pain.

    Includes index.
    1. Intractable pain—Treatment . 2. Intractable
pain—Psychological aspects.   I. Title. [DNLM:
1. Pain—psychology.   2. Pain—therapy.   WL 704 S839m]
RB127.S728   1987   616'.0472   86-25553
ISBN 0-399-13237-6

Typeset by Fisher Composition, Inc.

Printed in the United States of America
        2   3   4   5   6   7   8   9   10

FOR
JENNIFER & RUBÉN
AND DAVID

About the author

Dr. Richard A. Sternbach received his Ph.D. in psychology from UCLA in 1959 and has been a member of the medical school faculties of the University of Wisconsin, Madison, and the University of California, San Diego. His work in the theory and treatment of pain has received wide attention and is considered among the most innovative in the field. He has published over one hundred articles in various professional journals and written or edited an impressive list of books, including, *Pain: A Psychophysiological Analysis* (1968), *Pain Patients: Traits and Treatment* (1974) and *The Psychology of Pain* (1978). A founding member of the International Association for the Study of Pain and of the American Pain Society, he has received numerous research grants from the National Institute of Health. Since 1975 he has served as the director of the Pain Treatment Center at Scripps Clinic and Research Foundation at La Jolla, California, while continuing to give seminars on the treatment of pain to physicians and psychologists across the country and in much of Europe.

Contents

~~~~~~

Foreword

~~~~~~

This book contains a superb exposition of one of the most important and most pressing health-care problems in this and other industrialized nations—chronic pain. This importance stems from the fact that chronic pain afflicts about 30 percent of all Americans, and about one-half to two-thirds of these are either partially or totally disabled for periods of days, weeks and months, and some permanently. Consequently it is the most frequent cause of suffering and disability which impairs the quality of life of many individuals.

Dr. Sternbach, recognized worldwide as an outstanding authority on chronic pain, has done a remarkable job of presenting in this volume a comprehensive overview of various chronic-pain problems and how to cope with them. The book has been written in a very lucid, easily read and understood style and provides the reader with an excellent source of information on various aspects of pain and its treatment. In addition to the extremely well-written text, the book contains a number of highly instructive graphs and specific and poignant examples of how many of the author's patients cope with their pain. The entire book reflects an unusual degree of expertise and comprehensiveness and, most importantly, Dr. Sternbach's internationally known humaneness and intense interest in helping patients with chronic pain.

I recommend the book highly, not only to patients with chronic pain and their families, but also to the public as a whole because it will help people understand and appreciate the importance of this problem and how they can help afflicted friends cope with it. Indeed, I believe it will prove very useful to physicians and other health professionals who have the serious responsibility of caring for patients with chronic pain.

John J. Bonica, M.D., D.SC., FFARCS
Director Emeritus, Multidisciplinary Pain Center
University of Washington, Seattle

Preface

How can anyone live with pain? It robs us of sleep, drains us of energy, makes us irritable, prevents us from doing what we enjoy and leads us to feel despair. When pain lasts a long time, neurotic reactions are common. We show signs of depression, develop dependence on drugs and become preoccupied with the pain and other physical symptoms to the exclusion of almost everything else.

Pain is usually thought to be a warning signal, a symptom of an underlying disorder that needs to be treated. This is true of acute (short-lasting) pain, such as occurs with appendicitis, slipped disc or angina. But what of chronic (long-lasting) pain, which persists long after it has served its purpose? Then the pain itself is a problem and needs to be treated as a disease.

Physical conditioning and psychological training are the two main pillars of any pain treatment program. This book tells you about various methods of mastering chronic pain. Real patients, who have had severe pain of long duration, have learned to live satisfying lives despite pain by following these principles. Some learned to do this by themselves, some learned in pain treatment centers. It is they, really—the collective group of successful patients—who have written this book. Although their names are changed, the quotations attributed to them are their actual words, which illustrate what really worked for them. Combining their comments and supplementing them with my own observations from my experience in over fifteen years of practice with several thousands of chronic-pain patients, I have developed the principles of mastering chronic pain into a practical, effective 12-step program that you can use to help yourself with your pain problem and enable you to live—despite pain.

I have been doing research on pain since 1960 and working with pain patients since 1964. In 1975 I joined the Scripps Clinic and Research Foundation in La Jolla, California, as program director of the Pain Treatment Center. Through collaboration with Donald J. Dalessio, M.D., Chief of Medicine and one of the world's foremost authorities on headache, I have learned a great deal about this commonest of chronic-pain problems. In working with pain patients over the years, I have been impressed by the fact that successful patients have certain attitudes and techniques in common. Recently I contacted a number of the most successful of these patients and asked them to write their answers to the following: What philosophy, attitude or method of living with pain works for you? What do you do, and how?

In 1985 I had a chance to help design the first national survey on pain in the United States. This study was commissioned by the Bristol-Myers Company, the distributors of Nuprin, and it was conducted by Louis Harris & Associates, the national survey research organization, with whom I consulted. A representative sample of American adults was interviewed to learn how many had pain, what kinds of pain they had and what impact it had on their lives. The results were published in 1985 as The Nuprin Pain Report.

What was amazing to discover was how many Americans suffer pain. We learned that most persons had more than one kind of pain in the course of a year. Some 73 percent of adults (127 million) had one or more headaches in the previous year. More than 56 percent (97.4 million) had back pains, 53 percent (97.2 million) had muscle pains, 51 percent (88.7 million) had joint pains, etc.

Worse still, 12.8 percent, or 20.8 million adults, reported *chronic* pain, which they had had at least 101 days during the preceding year. All persons with pain report that it disrupts their lives. It interferes with their daily routines, disrupts their being able to concentrate on their work or to enjoy leisure activities.

As if the extent of suffering due to pain was not enough, the economic consequences are enormous. In our survey, the *average* individual adult lost about 23 days a year due to a pain problem. Of those working at full-time jobs, 5 work days per year were lost, for a total of 550 million work days lost in one year alone because of pain. This amounts to $55 billion per year of lost productivity!

If we add to this the loss of productivity of part-time workers and the costs of disability payments to those unable to work because of pain-related problems, the cost to our economy is probably close to an appalling *$80 billion per year!*

This book is an outgrowth of a booklet I wrote that appeared in 1977 and, in a revised edition, 1983. Those booklets were sold at cost to pain clinics around the United States for distribution to their patients. Over the years, several thousands of copies have been distributed.

This is the first book, to my knowledge, that tells you in a systematic way what you can do to master your pain. Most of you will be able to read it and master pain yourselves, but some may need the assistance of a pain treatment program. For the latter group, this book will be a guide, explaining what to expect and offering a standard by which to evaluate programs.

For both groups, however, this book should show that it is indeed possible to master pain, and to point the way. The steps listed below are a summary of the principles described in the following chapters.

1. Accept the fact of having chronic pain.

2. Set specific goals for work, hobbies and social activities toward which you will work.

3. Let yourself get angry at your pain if it seems to be getting the best of you.

4. Take your analgesics on a strict time schedule, and then taper off until you are no longer taking any.

5. Get in the best physical shape possible, and keep fit.

6. Learn how to relax, and practice relaxation techniques regularly.

7. Keep yourself busy.

8. Pace your activities.

9. Have your family and friends support only your healthy behavior, not your invalidism.

10. Be open and reasonable with your doctor.

11. Practice effective empathy with others having pain problems.

12. Remain hopeful.

If you follow these twelve steps you can expect to control your chronic pain better than you ever thought you could.

1.
The Chronic-Pain Problem

It is not true that suffering ennobles the character; happiness does that sometimes, but suffering, for the most part, makes men petty and vindictive.

W. Somerset Maugham

I can see what Nancy's pain problem is as she comes into my office. She is about 40 years old, looks pale and carries herself very stiffly. She turns her entire upper body instead of just her head. She holds her neck rigid, and her teeth are clenched when she says hello.

"Have you been having headaches for a long time?" I ask, after we sit down.

"Ever since the accident. I was stopped at a signal and a pickup truck going about 45 rear-ended me. That was three years ago."

"What are the headaches like? What do they feel like?"

"It's like my head's in a vise. It starts in my neck and goes up the back of my head and runs all the way around. I have it when I wake up in the morning and when I go to bed at night. There's never a time when I'm free of it. Sometimes it's so bad I can hardly see. And sometimes my neck feels so weak that I can hardly hold my head up."

So far, this is all a classical history for a tension (muscle-contraction) headache and neck pain. Now I need to learn why she hasn't recovered yet.

"What have you tried to help it?"

"I had physical therapy for three months. Ultrasound and moist heat and massage. Then I tried acupuncture and then I went to a chiropractor. And I tried every kind of muscle relaxer you could think of. They helped at first, but I couldn't do anything but sleep, so I had to stop using them."

"What are you using now?"

"I'm taking Darvocet, eight a day. I have to take two at a time. Even so, they don't help that much."

She's very concise in her answers, no long-winded dramatic stories, no defensive self-justification. I notice again how tight her muscles are.

"Do you happen to notice if you grind your teeth at night? Or has your dentist mentioned anything about it?"

"I think I must. Sometimes my teeth hurt in the morning. And my dentist says it looks like I'm wearing them down. But I don't even know when I'm doing it."

She's honest in admitting to doing something that could be contributing to her pain. Most people find it hard to recognize the role they play in their problem. They don't like to hear about "tension headache" or "nerves" or "stress." They think it's like saying that their pain is imaginary or that they're making it up.

But Nancy seems willing to consider anything that sheds light on the problem. She hasn't closed her mind to anything about the pain.

"It must be really hard, hurting like this for such a long time."

She doesn't say anything, but her eyes fill with tears. I push the box of tissues across the desk toward her.

"I wasn't going to do this," she says, angry with herself as she snatches tissues and dabs at her eyes.

I look out the window as she cries a little bit and blows her nose. I don't know how many times I've heard this story. Hundreds, at least. None of these people know each other, although they could form a "whiplash club," so similar are their stories. If I added those whose pain started with some other kind of stress or injury but which also continued past the point of healing due to chronic muscle contraction—there must have been thousands of them.

"Okay," I tell her, "what's been the effect of the pain on your life?"

In the next half-hour more tissues are used as she tells me how she's had to take a medical leave from her job because she was missing too many days' work due to splitting headaches. Her children avoid her because of her irritable temper. She and her husband rarely go out now, never have guests over, because she simply doesn't feel up to it.

For three years she's been unable to function normally. She feels increasingly disabled, barely able to keep up with minimal housework, feeling ill with the pain of the headache and from the pain pills. She has no energy, feels tired all the time and cries a lot. She thinks she has become depressed because of this.

Nancy's story is mirrored by those of millions of persons with headache, back pain, abdominal pain, arthritis, neuralgia, etc. Her treatment began routinely and proceeded without a problem. She had biofeedback training to learn cervical and scalp muscle-relaxation techniques, and physical-therapy stretching exercises and aerobics conditioning to help discharge muscle tension. She gave up caffeine, which was contributing to the irritability of the muscle fibers and their sustained contraction.

Nancy was faithful about attending the biofeedback and physical-therapy sessions, practicing the techniques several times daily at home, as instructed.

"I came here to get better," she said, "and that's my priority. I'd be foolish not to work at this."

"Well," I said, "I did warn you that it would take most of your time each day for a couple of months. But I'm impressed with how well you're doing."

Nancy flashed a big smile. "I haven't had a headache for three days now, and I've only been at this for two weeks. And I'm down to only two Darvocet a day. I have to admit I was pretty skeptical at first, but I'm a believer now. That biofeedback machine showed me that I wasn't really relaxing when I thought I was. It's amazing how you can fool yourself. But now I can tell when I start tensing up and catch myself before I get a headache. What a difference!"

In just two more weeks Nancy was discharged from this outpatient program, to return in one month for a follow-up evaluation. She was entirely free of headaches and seemed a much brighter and more cheerful person.

"This is the real me you're seeing now," she said. "I feel like a cloud has been lifted off my mind. I didn't realize what a fog I was living in with all that pain and the pain pills I was taking. Now I feel like I'm living again. You tell all the other patients that this really works. Tell them that if they do what they're supposed to, they can get better. They may have nerve damage or whatever, and still have some pain, but they can get better. Just tell them that."

What Chronic Pain Does to Us
Probably the commonest complaint of those with chronic pain is that their sleep is disturbed. Before the pain began, they always slept well. Since the pain developed, they have trouble

falling asleep because they cannot get comfortable. As they finally settle into a less uncomfortable position, they find the pain becoming more prominent in their minds as there is less to distract them. Finally, exhausted, they drift into a restless sleep, only to awaken every hour or so as they roll over or change position and the pain awakens them.

They finally remain awake until three or four in the morning, unable to get back to sleep, and at such times find it impossible not to think about what the pain means—whether the doctors have made an incorrect diagnosis or are keeping some terrible secret, whether it is worth trying to go on living with such pain, whether there is any other way out.

Even the minority who are able to sleep well report that they feel quite exhausted all the time, drained of energy as though they had the flu. The continuous pain wears them down. If, in addition to this fatigue, there is the disturbance of sleep, the people feel even less able to bear the pain; indeed, they become less tolerant of any pain. Even minor injuries, such as those caused by bumping into a piece of furniture or stubbing a toe, seem like major calamities.

Usually those with chronic pain are taking analgesics. One of the side effects of such drugs is to upset the stomach and gut. Patients frequently complain of heartburn and constipation, feeling nauseated and bilious. They find the analgesics becoming less effective over time; they need to take larger amounts just to "take the edge off" the pain, and so still more severe side effects develop.

How miserable these people feel. In addition to being in pain, they are tired all the time, they cannot sleep and their bowels don't function properly. And yet these physical problems are only part of the chronic-pain syndrome. There are psychological effects too.

Those with chronic pain complain of having become very

irritable and short-tempered. They find themselves flaring up in anger over the minor actions and trivial comments of those around them. They say hurtful things to family members for insufficient reasons, then feel guilty and promise to keep their tempers and hold their tongues, only to lose control again and again. They then begin to seclude themselves to avoid further attacking those they are close to. They thus find themselves withdrawing more and more, often becoming almost home-bound, sometimes even spending most of the time in the bed-room, alone, with little to distract them from their pain.

Some persons with chronic pain feel so nauseated by their pain and analgesics that they lose their appetites, need to force themselves to eat a minimum amount of food and slowly but steadily lose weight. Others find themselves restless and on edge and do a great deal of nervous snacking and excessive eating. This, combined with their inactivity, causes them to steadily gain weight, often becoming somewhat obese, and to become disgusted with themselves.

The disturbances of sleep and appetite and the resulting social withdrawal are some of the elements underlying depression. Almost all reports of psychiatric and psychological studies of chronic-pain patients report significant depression as one of the results. It is not exactly the same as the kind of depression that psychiatric patients show, but it is a depression nevertheless. Some of the persons with chronic pain admit to feeling depressed, but many do not, insisting that it is pain and not depression that spoils their sleep, makes them withdraw and so on.

In addition to this kind of depression, many of those with chronic pain begin to think of themselves as chronic invalids or, at least, chronically disabled. They are often unable to continue working, and receive disability or workers' compensation income, which only partly compensates for the lost salary or wages, and this begins to contribute to a shift in the family dynamics and power structure.

With one of the wage earners unable to bring in the accustomed income, unable to help with the household chores and more and more withdrawn, the center of the family shifts away from the person with pain to those who are more active and involved, and the patient becomes (and feels) less important. The other family members, for their part, feel sorry for the one with pain, frustrated and guilty because they cannot help relieve the pain and—so secretly that they hardly admit it to themselves—somewhat resentful that they have to do more chores now.

Some families remain in this state of strain and tension. In others, the patient begins to lose his or her sense of status and, without realizing it, begins to tyrannize the family. This may occur directly, through irritability and temper outbursts, or indirectly, through manipulating others to do things the person could do for himself or herself. These manipulations are made possible through the guilt feelings of the family members, who are powerless to help the sufferer and resent his or her disability.

The physical problems (sleep disturbance, appetite disturbance, fatigue, etc.) and psychological problems (irritability, depression, social withdrawal) and family problems are serious enough, but that is not all there is to the chronic-pain syndrome. There are serious problems as well with doctors, with the health-care system and with the insurance and disability systems.

The person with chronic pain usually has a much higher proportion of medical contacts than do other patients. Because, despite the patient's insistent requests, the physician cannot provide relief, the patient may begin soliciting help from other physicians, requesting intervention in the form of surgery or analgesic prescriptions. The doctors become frustrated because their ability to cure or at least provide relief is stymied, and they begin to wonder whether the patient is or will become a drug addict, or whether psychological symptoms may be causing the pain. The patient and physician become increasingly irritated and frustrated with each other, and mutual suspicion begins to develop.

Partly in desperation, partly because of hope, the patient begins to try alternative health-care systems. Various forms of massage and manipulation, nutritional plans and food supplements are tried, with some possible slight but temporary improvement noted. As the patient reports this to his or her doctor, the physician becomes more annoyed, and notes about the patient's emotional problems and drug use become more prominent in the record. The medical-insurance or health-plan system begins not only to refuse reimbursement for the nontraditional treatments the patient has received, but to question the need for even the more orthodox medical treatments.

Many patients begin to find that much of their time is spent filling out claim forms. Not only are requests for reimbursement of medical expenses slow in being filled, but more and more of them are being denied and must be appealed. Disability checks suddenly stop arriving, without explanation, and the patient learns only weeks or months later that this is due to a casual comment by one or another physician to the effect that she or he does not think the patient is really all that disabled, and that psychological factors seem to be prominent in the case. Some patients find themselves being followed and photographed by insurance investigators who are hired to take films of the patient to prove that he or she is not really disabled. The patient becomes increasingly angry and embittered and—like it or not—poorer.

The chronic-pain syndrome consists of the physical, mental, familial and social problems we have just described. These are not imaginary. They do not cause the pain, but they certainly make the pain seem worse and harder to deal with. They do cause *excessive* pain and *excessive* disability. We will deal with these problems specifically and in some detail in later chapters. At this point we are only mentioning them to give an idea of the extent of the problem and to help you to realize that the problems you may have encountered are not unique, but are well known. And furthermore, there are specific ways of dealing with them that make it possible to have better means of pain control and to live a more satisfying life.

But the effects of chronic pain on the individual and the family and on social contacts are still only part of the story. There are many such individuals, and when the total costs of acute and chronic pain are estimated, they are truly staggering.

What Is Pain?
Each of us believes that we know, from our own experiences, what pain is. But different persons have different experiences, and the word "pain" may mean something different to each one of us. The following definition is the one adopted by the International Association for the Study of Pain.

Pain is an unpleasant sensory and emotional experience associated with actual or potential tissue damage, or described in terms of such damage. Pain is always subjective, an experience. There is no method now available for measuring pain in a purely objective manner—the way a thermometer can be used to measure body temperature. We rely on the individual to tell us or show us in some way that pain is being experienced.

Because pain is always unpleasant, it is not merely a sensation from a certain part of the body, but also an emotional experience. The things that cause pain are those which are likely to cause damage to the body, or nearly so, and we feel those sensations, but there is also an accompanying emotional experience.

It has become fashionable in certain circles to refer to such emotional distress as grief, loneliness, anger, etc., as "pain," as in, "His wife left him, and he has to share that pain with someone." This is using the word pain as a metaphor. Some emotions may be painful, but they are not pain. We will be using the word pain to refer to the unpleasant *physical* sensations and accompanying emotional experiences associated with tissue damage.

Some persons report pain with no apparent injury nor any physiological cause for it. After appropriate studies, it usually turns out that this is due to psychological causes. Yet their experience of pain is the same as that of those whose pain is due to physical injury, judging by their reports of what they feel, since they describe it in terms of tissue damage. Although we accept their experience as pain, this book is written primarily for those whose pain is associated with actual damage, and which persists. But we discuss psychologically caused pain in another chapter.

Acute Pain, Chronic Pain

Acute pain refers to pain of recent onset or short duration. It is experienced when we stub a bare toe against a rock, or are sunburned, or have a headache, or sprain our back, and so on. Acute pain also occurs with gallstones or kidney stones, heart attacks and many other diseases.

In each of these conditions, some injury is occurring, or changes are beginning that could lead to injury if increased or continued for long. In this sense, *pain may be a warning signal* to avoid further damage or to seek help.

In some cases, however, the warning signal comes too late to avoid injury. A severe sunburn is a good example—we do not feel the pain until after the too-lengthy exposure to the sun has occurred. Similarly, there are many instances of injuries that are painless when they happen, as in wounds or the neck muscle strain that comes with a "whiplash" injury, but which are followed by pain some hours or days later. In these cases, *pain may be a special "need-state"* meant to keep us still so that healing can occur.

When acute pain occurs, the emotion which accompanies it is very similar to anxiety. We feel apprehensive about the pain itself and whether it will become worse, and we are worried about what the injury or disease means with respect to our health and ability to function. This anxiety is not likely to amount to much if the pain is one we understand, such as the stubbed toe or sunburn; but the anxiety can be quite great if the pain is both severe and one we do not understand, such as sudden pain in the chest or belly.

Emotions such as anxiety have bodily components as well as our mental experience of them. In both anxiety and acute pain, there may occur increases in heart rate, blood pressure, rate of breathing, sweating and muscle tension as the body mobilizes for an emergency. These bodily changes can even become conditioned to the entire situation around the painful experience, so that we begin to experience them in anticipation of pain. This can occur, for example, as we prepare for a needle stick for blood drawing or as we enter a dental suite. We can observe it in young children returning to the pediatric office, or pets being brought back to the veterinarian's office— the cries and struggles which originally followed the experience of pain have been so conditioned that they now occur in anticipation of it.

The connection between anxiety and acute pain has been studied a great deal. It has been found that patients who appear to be more anxious on psychological tests usually have more pain and slower recovery after surgery than those who are less anxious. And treating those with acute pain with an antianxiety medication tends to reduce the severity of pain and makes pain control possible with smaller amounts of analgesics.

In general, acute pain is well understood and well managed in medical settings. Trivial everyday events, such as sunburn, tension headache and stubbed toe, most of us can manage ourselves, but we could be concerned about, even frightened by, very severe pains which develop quickly or even suddenly, and which we do not understand. Trauma centers and emergency rooms are well equipped to deal with these problems. Analgesics are given immediately, and diagnostic and treatment measures are taken at once to identify and resolve the cause of the pain. Almost always, in acute situations, *the pain is most appropriately thought of as a symptom* of some underlying problem that needs to be found and treated, and modern techniques for doing so are remarkably effective.

But what of the situation where pain is persistent? Pain may develop slowly and gradually, as in some cases of back problems, of aching joints or of adhesions following surgery. Or pain may develop suddenly following an injury or disease and simply persist indefinitely, long after the healing process has taken place. This can occur because permanent damage to some tissue has occurred, including possible scarring along nerve endings or pathways, or the kinds of damage to joints that occur with arthritis.

This persistence of pain is called chronic pain. Chronic pain exists when an acute-pain problem has stabilized, that is, further healing is not likely to occur and there is not likely to be any change in the intensity of the pain itself. As a rule of thumb, any pain that persists for more than three to six months may be considered chronic.

As with acute pain, chronic pain may vary in intensity from very mild or slight to very severe or unbearable. It may vary from day to day, or even throughout the day. Some persons may have only a mildly nagging ache, which they forget about most of the time and hesitate even to call pain. Others have daily pain so intense as to make them incapable of functioning.

Just as the intensity of pain varies, so does its time course. For some, the pain is constant, never varying. For others, the pain varies depending upon their position or activity. For still others, the pain changes unpredictably, unrelated to anything the individual can identify.

In almost all cases of chronic pain, the underlying cause of the pain has been identified and treated, but the pain persists. In cases of trauma or postoperative pain, healing has occurred but the pain continues. In cases of disease, the underlying problem has been (or is being) treated, but pain remains a problem—for example, in arthritis, diabetes, cancer, etc. The point of repeating this is to emphasize something that is often overlooked—the very important differences between acute and chronic pain. These are more than just the difference between short-term and long-term pain.

Unlike acute pain,

- chronic pain is not a symptom;
- chronic pain is not a warning signal;
- chronic pain is not a need-state for rest.

Chronic pain is a syndrome composed of a number of physical, emotional and behavioral changes which can convert otherwise healthy persons into invalids. Chronic pain is like a "false alarm"—a warning signal that serves no purpose. In its effect on the individual who has it and on the family, chronic pain is very like a debilitating disease.

Does Pain Ennoble the Spirit?

There is an old religious point of view which holds that pain and suffering are good because they purify the soul; the sense of pain was given us so that we could learn to ignore the needs of the body and put our minds on spiritual things. Only the pure would enter heaven, and so pain served the purpose of destroying lower animal instincts and pleasures. This argument was used by those religious authorities who tortured others and by some religious groups who inflicted pain on themselves. Some writers in this century have even perpetuated this old idea.

I am unaware of any evidence that can support this argument. It is apparently one of those ideas that sounds as though it were plausible, but really has no basis in fact. It is conceivable that a brief episode of pain might make a person more sympathetic toward others who have pain, but chronic pain appears to be absolutely destructive, with few exceptions. We will simply mention here that numerous studies of persons with chronic pain show that it has a destructive effect on the body, on the emotions, on daily functioning. More than one person has committed suicide because of pain that could not be tolerated. More than one family has been broken by the devastating impact of chronic pain on one of its members. Whether the suicide or the broken family had purified souls as a result of the pain experience is impossible to know, but their lives were certainly made wretched.

The idea that we are born to have pain and therefore it is good for us was used by both medical and religious spokesmen of the last century, after the discovery of anesthesia, to oppose its use for surgery and labor. They actually argued that God meant us to have pain and to suffer and that anesthesia and analgesia should not be permitted. Fortunately for us they did not prevail, perhaps because they had no answer for those who wondered why God permitted the discovery of the means to pain relief.

It is a commonsense observation that severe pain of long duration has a destructive effect on all aspects of the individual—this is the basis for torture. Studies of individuals who have been through extended periods of torture show that the effects are quite similar to those who have had severe chronic pain due to disease or injury—and the effects are all negative, so far as we can judge, and from what the victims themselves say.

2.
How Pain Works

In this chapter we describe the pain system and how it works. It is important to bear in mind that the more you understand about how the pain system is organized, the less you need be frightened by the pain and the better you will be able to understand the reasons for the pain-control techniques that are described in this book. Although the simple descriptions given here will not make you a medical expert on pain, they may be enable you to understand better the physicians who are consulted about the pain problem.

Pain Receptors

The nerve endings that detect damage or potential damage to the body are described as "free nerve endings" because of their appearance under the microscope. They are called nociceptors, or pain receptors, because of their function—they are the sensors that detect the changes in the body which, when the signals reach the brain, will be felt as pain.

There are three kinds of pain receptors. One responds only

to a great deal of force, such as a blow, or pressure. Another responds only to heat above a certain temperature, and a third kind responds to varying degrees of pressure and temperature and chemical changes around the nerve endings. The last two kinds, the heat pain receptors and the "wide dynamic range" pain receptors, can be sensitized as the nerves regrow after an injury. This sensitization means that they can be made to respond with an injury signal even to things that do not threaten damage, such as light touch or pressure. This sensitization occurs in pain conditions following burns or nerve injuries.

Pain Pathways

There are two kinds of nerve fibers that conduct the injury signals from the pain receptors to the first relay in the spinal cord. The thinnest of all the nerve fibers conduct signals that will be perceived as slow, aching, burning and long-lasting pain, not precisely located in the body. These are called C fibers, and transmit most of the injury signals that lead to the troublesome pain problems encountered in pain clinics. The other nerve fibers, called A-delta, are slightly thicker and transmit injury signals that are fast, sharp and well localized. These are the kind of pain we feel more often in acute-pain states, when we are injured, for example.

There is a relay in the spinal cord where nerve fibers from all parts of the body end and connect to the next set of pathways. The nerve fibers collect in the spinal cord, entering it at different levels. Thus, signals coming from the feet and legs are transmitted first to the lower part of the spine, those from the arms and neck to the topmost part. They join with other fibers in bundles, called tracts, within the spinal cord and, just above it, in the brain stem, like small streams merging into a river.

When they are collected in the spinal cord, most of the connecting fibers cross over to the opposite side and proceed toward the brain; about 70–80 percent of the injury signals cross in this way. That is why, if a person has a stroke or other damage to, say, the right side of the brain, it is the left side of the body that feels "dead" or numb.

There are two main routes that the injury signals take on their way to the brain. One, which apparently developed first in the course of evolution, is called the paleospinothalamic tract and runs along the center of the spinal cord. Paleo means old, and spinothalamic means that the pathway conducts injury signals from the spine to the part of the midbrain called the thalamus. The fibers in this pathway make many connections, and the signals are conducted relatively slowly. The information transmitted along this system is of deep, burning, aching pain, often imprecisely localized.

The other major route for injury signals in the spinal cord is the neospinothalamic tract, so called because it is newer, that is, developed later in the evolutionary process. It carries more information and does so more efficiently. There are few connections, and the fibers conduct signals more rapidly, so that the injury signals arrive in the brain quickly. The pain is more precisely localized and is felt as sharp and intense.

All along the pathways to the brain, information is sent off in various directions about the injury signal itself. Even at the first relay in the spinal cord, connections are made sending messages directly to the muscles to cause the person to jerk away from the source of injury. And other signals are sent off that cause the heart to pound, blood pressure to increase, the lungs to take in more oxygen, the pupils to dilate (to see more clearly), the blood to receive more sugar and adrenaline for energy and the entire brain to become more aroused and alert—all this in addition to the actual processing of the injury signal itself.

We have been using the term "injury signal" up to this point, because the messages that have gone off in all directions to the various body parts have been about the injury only. The signals are not felt as "pain" until they reach the brain. Even though we feel the pain in the foot or the back or wherever the injury is, the "feeling" actually occurs in the brain. To paraphrase the line in *My Fair Lady*, "The reign of pain is mainly in the brain."

Although there does not seem to be a precise "pain center" in the brain, it does seem as if injury signals become pain signals when they arrive at the thalamus, a structure deep in the middle of the brain. But things do not stop here. The journey from the injured part to the spinal cord and on through brain stem to the thalamus, with collateral signals going off in all directions, takes just a fraction of a second and yet is only about half of the process.

From the thalamus, relays are made to the outer part of the brain called the sensory cortex. Here we receive specific information about the pain—where it is, what kind of pain, etc. But now also a most surprising thing happens. Even as pain signals are occurring in the thalamus, damping signals are sent back down the spinal cord to raise the threshold of the cells there to incoming injury signals. A process much like automatic gain control occurs, limiting the amount of pain we experience. It has been called a gate control process. Although we may feel that our pain is (or has been) as intense as we could possibly stand, nevertheless it could be far worse if these damping signals were not automatically sent back down to the spinal cord.

These damping signals cause the first relay cells in the spinal cord to resist reacting to incoming injury signals, and so fewer messages about the injury are sent on to the brain. Thus, the first signals of pain start a sequence of events which, like automatic gain control or negative feedback, reduce the number of injury signals that reach the thalamus, and thus, supposedly, the experience of pain is less intense.

There are several things in addition to pain that can raise the pain threshold in this way. Stress of various kinds, exercise and intense but nonpainful stimulation can all produce this effect. This information is of practical value to those with chronic pain as it is the basis for techniques utilized in a "natural" and nonharmful approach to pain control. We will describe these techniques in detail in later chapters.

Some Pain Chemistry

There are areas of the brain and brain stem that can be given very weak electrical stimulation, and which then activate the descending gate control system. These areas are the same sites that contain opiate receptors, places on cells that react to narcotic analgesics such as morphine. The nervous system has its own analgesics, which are called into play when pain occurs, and these seem to be a part of the gate control mechanism.

Endorphins, enkephalins and dynorphin are some of the pain-suppressing chemicals that have been found, and there are probably others as well. Different kinds of opiate receptors have also been found that are unlike those which are sensitive to morphine. This gives hope that entirely new kinds of analgesics may be synthesized one day that will not have the drawbacks and side effects which complicate the use of analgesics today.

There is another gate control process that does not seem to rely on an opiate circuit. It continues to operate even when opiates are blocked by giving narcotic antagonists. This component of the descending inhibitory system uses a different process to send the signals down to the spinal cord—one of its chemicals is serotonin. Serotonin, which has a different role in different parts of the body, is a very interesting and important chemical. In the brain it seems essential for sleep and for emotional balance. When serotonin is depleted, insomnia and depression result—and, apparently, a decrease in tolerance for pain.

It seems as though some of the characteristics of the chronic-pain syndrome—sleep disturbance, irritability, depression and lessened tolerance for pain—could be explained by abnormally low levels of brain serotonin. This is not proved and still speculative, but it is possible that long-lasting pain may result in decreased brain serotonin, accounting for the changes observed in the chronic-pain syndrome. It is certainly true that medications which work to increase brain serotonin activity have reversed the symptoms of the chronic-pain syndrome for many thousands of patients (but not all), improving sleep, alleviating depression and reducing somewhat the severity of their pain. We will discuss this method of managing chronic pain in a later chapter.

A "Simple" Solution

Many persons have the idea that the pain system works like a telephone line: an injury signal starts at one end and travels along the nerve to the other end, where a bell rings to signal "pain." In this model, it would be an obvious conclusion that, to stop pain, one should simply cut the nerve. This does not work for chronic pain, however, and we will discuss surgical approaches, as well as others, in Chapter 4.

We have already indicated that there is a two-way communication in the pain system. There are at least two major inputs and two major descending pain-control systems. Cutting pain pathways can destroy the latter as well as the former, so that in some cases the pain is actually made worse.

We also mentioned that when injury signals enter the spinal cord, most of the relays then cross to the other side. But not all of them do: some 20–30 percent travel to the brain on the same side. This makes it very nearly impossible to cut out all the signals going to the brain to be felt as pain.

In addition, there is a great deal of overlap and redundancy in the nervous system. The pain receptors, for example, are densely packed together, and any natural injury (a blow or a burn, for example) stimulates thousands of them. Many nerve fibers are involved, and they enter the spinal cord at several different levels. And, as mentioned earlier, their injury or alarm signals go off in a number of directions to different body systems, in addition to signaling "pain" in the thalamus, in order to prepare the body to survive the threat.

All of this overlap and redundancy suggests that pain is a very primitive sense which is built into our bodies to ensure our ability to survive. If pain were eliminated completely after a single blow or wound, our survival would be easily threatened; so in the course of evolution, we developed several overlapping pain systems, which enhance our ability to avoid or escape injurious stimulation and promote healing if injury occurs.

Although it is disappointing to many who suffer long-standing severe pain, it does not now seem possible to make a simple cut of a nerve or nerve pathway to eliminate pain in a part of the body—not for the long run, and not without causing many complications, such as numbness and weakness and uselessness of the body part, and not without the possibility of pain returning.

Insensitivity to Pain
We can appreciate the importance of the sense of pain by seeing what happens to those who lose it—or are born without it. There are some individuals who suffer nerve damage due to disease, such as diabetes or a viral infection such as shingles

(herpes zoster), or because of injury or, on occasion, because of surgery. Such persons have a very difficult time properly caring for the involved area because they do not feel pain there. It is not uncommon for a sore on the foot, for example, to become badly infected without the person realizing it, and often an amputation is necessary as a lifesaving measure.

Similarly, some individuals have lost the sense of pain in an eye, due to shingles or a surgical procedure, and consequently fail to be aware of irritations to the eye, do not blink automatically to produce more tears and therefore suffer abrasions and scarring to the cornea with resultant impaired vision.

Even more dramatic consequences occur to those born insensitive to pain. Such persons are quite rare, especially those who are normal in all other respects (not brain damaged nor severely retarded). The infants and young children injure themselves repeatedly—it does not hurt them to jump from heights, or fall, or burn themselves, and many die young from trauma or infections. They have no pain symptoms from broken ankles or feet, they have no "stomachache" from appendicitis, etc. Severe degenerative changes and inflammations result from repeated trauma, even from such simple things as sitting in one position too long without feeling uncomfortable and moving around.

It is not clear exactly what the physical basis is for lack of the sense of pain in those who are normal in every other respect. They are certainly not mentally or emotionally disturbed—not those who survived to adulthood and were studied, at any rate. The best hypothesis is that such individuals have either an excess of brain enkephalins or endorphins, or a deficit of substance P—a chemical involved in the transmission of injury signals in the spinal cord. In any case, such rare individuals show us clearly how essential pain is to a healthy life, and despite the problems of managing chronic pain, an attempt to eliminate the sense of pain completely is probably not the answer (even if it were possible), because its elimination causes many more problems than it solves.

Phantom Limb Pain

Another kind of problem altogether is that of individuals who have pain in an arm or leg that has been amputated. Those who are born with missing limbs never have such sensations. But those who have a limb amputated after early childhood almost always experience feelings in the missing part, which disappear only slowly and gradually over a period of months.

A small percentage—perhaps 10 percent—experience not only sensations in general, but pain in particular, and if the pain persists, the phantom sensations (the feelings that the missing part is still there) do not disappear. Usually the pain is felt exactly as it was before the amputation—as from a crushed foot, for example, or a burned arm. And the pain usually is constant, although sometimes it comes and goes in an unpredictable way.

Such individuals also are not mentally or emotionally disturbed, and they are not imagining their pain. In a few cases they may have neuromas in the stump—tender spots due to scarring of nerve endings—but these are not usually related to the phantom pain, and in any event, most phantom limb pain occurs without such neuromas being present.

What these cases teach us is that pain can become centralized. When leg or arm pain continues for a while, and then the limb is amputated, the injury signals continue being generated in the spinal cord, brain stem and brain, causing the pain to continue to be felt as it was before. This effect is enhanced by the fact that there are now no other sensations coming from the missing limb to stop these injury signals, to "tell" the brain that the source of pain is gone.

It is not clear why some individuals develop phantom limb pain and some do not. Fortunately, those who do can benefit a great deal from stimulation techniques, described in another chapter, which seem to interrupt the centralized pain and "tell" the brain that there is no pain in that limb.

Many persons with chronic pain, especially when it is localized in an arm or leg, wish at times that someone would just cut the thing off and be done with it. These cases of phantom limb pain teach us that this approach would not necessarily be successful. And when the source of the pain is in the spine, for example in chronic disc problems with pain going into the limb, or referred from the brain (after a stroke), then of course amputation will not help at all.

Modulating Pain

In many cases it is simply not possible to correct the physical problem causing the chronic pain. Usually one cannot simply cut out the pain with any surgical procedure. This is because of the overlapping and redundant inputs of injury signals, because continued pain may result because it has become centralized, and because of other unacceptable consequences of such surgery, which will be discussed later. Many different surgical approaches have been tried over the years and found to have an unsatisfactory success rate over the long run.

Although chronic pain may not usually be eliminated, it most certainly can be modulated. It can be reduced to an acceptable or tolerable level, and individuals can learn how to get on with their lives despite the remaining pain.

3.
Attitudes
Toward Pain

Those who have trouble mastering pain usually have wrong ideas about the meaning of their pain, or attitudes about it that get in the way of overcoming it. In working with thousands of pain patients over the years, I noticed that those who are successful in coping with pain have certain attitudes in common. So, recently, I made a point of asking a number of them to write their answers to these questions: What philosophy, attitude or method of living with pain works for you? What do you do, and how?

They were pleased and eager to answer, hoping that their experiences would help others. I combined their comments with my own observations, and certain common ideas emerged consistently. I found that whenever a pain patient incorporates these ideas into his or her life, the mastery of chronic pain comes along rapidly.

If you have a defeatist attitude, or believe that you are still "sick" or an invalid, you will simply go through the motions of getting better and remain as disabled as before.

In this chapter I describe some attitudes that are basic to learning to live with pain successfully. You may already have these attitudes and simply need to apply the techniques described in subsequent chapters. Or you may need to consider seriously these ideas and make some changes in your thinking. These attitudes include realistic acceptance of having pain; setting goals involving specific achievements in the areas of work, recreation and social activities; expressing anger appropriately and remaining optimistic about getting on with the business of living.

Realistic Acceptance

There are some pains for which there is no relief available yet. That is a fact. There is no "cure" for some chronic pains.

If you have chronic pain, and several reputable physicians and consultants have indicated that there is no remedy for it, you must accept that fact. You should not go doctor-shopping, looking for a miracle. There are some conditions, such as arthritis, degenerative spine disease, peripheral nerve damage, "thalamic pain" (following a stroke), etc., that are going to continue causing pain.

The Wrong Attitude

Sam is a 46-year-old Oklahoman who has had three back operations. For twenty years he has been operating bulldozers and Caterpillar tractors during the week and following the rodeo circuit on weekends as a contestant in bronc and steer riding. He has earned big wages as an "operating engineer" in construction work and many rodeo prizes. But his spine has taken a terrible pounding in both activities. As he stands in my office (he is too uncomfortable to sit), I notice his belt buckle, which says, "All-Around Champion, 1970."

Sam apologizes for standing, but says his back hurts too much to sit. He is 6 feet tall, about 180 pounds, and despite much forced inactivity for the past year, he is as hard muscled and trim as a young athlete. He briefly describes his accident, the surgery he has had to remove discs and to fuse his spine, and tells how he has refused all analgesics despite pain so severe he could barely drive his pickup truck to our clinic.

Sam limps slowly back and forth in my office as he comes to the point of his visit. "When I went back to the doc that operated on me, he said that there was nothing more he could do and I'd have to learn to live with the pain." Sam's jaw muscles twitch as he blurts out angrily, "Now that's a helluva thing for a doctor to say! I think it's a stupid thing to say. I'm going to get rid of this pain!"

"Suppose," I ask, "we can't take away your pain?"

Sam looks at me for a moment. "Then I'll find someone who will," he says. "I don't give up easy."

Sam could be headed for big trouble, if he turns his determination and toughness to the task of finding someone to remove his pain. He might find someone who will try and almost certainly fail, leaving him crippled and with more pain than before.

By using the word "acceptance," we mean accepting the *fact* of having pain that is not going to go away. This does *not* mean having to like it, or giving in to it and becoming an invalid. Rather, it means deciding that nothing more can be done, medically or surgically, to eliminate the pain—and then going on from there.

At what point should a person decide to accept the pain and give up trying to find a cure? There is no precise answer to this because it depends upon the kind of pain problem and how severe it is and the kinds of doctors consulted.

I have known persons who had a quite mild pain, such as stiffness of the back, who actually launched themselves into a full career as "professional pain patients," determined to find a diagnosis and cure. They gave up their jobs, took a small amount of disability income and spent their time going to doctors and clinics to get a diagnosis. They had never had back pain before and, for one reason or another, experiencing the pain was very upsetting. They worried about what the pain meant. They couldn't believe it was not a warning signal of some serious disease. When all examinations showed nothing abnormal, they would go off somewhere else to have further evaluations. They refused all treatment because they didn't want the symptoms "covered up." Although they probably had chronic strain, which could be successfully relieved, and although the pain was really mild and not disabling, the campaign to find a serious diagnosis (which could not succeed) displaced all other purposes in their lives.

The Right Attitude

Fred is a 53-year-old meat broker. Twenty years ago he was a butcher, lifting and carrying and chopping up 100-pound sides of beef all day. He suffered a ruptured disk, had it removed and developed a staph infection in the incision. For eighteen months he remained in the hospital and had several operations to drain the infection. Finally, he was discharged with arachnoiditis, a chronic scarring of the nerves in the spine, which left him with severe back and leg pain. Unable to return to his trade, he used his knowledge of meats to get into the wholesale and brokerage business.

Like Sam, Fred also prefers to stay on his feet in the office. He is a grizzled, tough-talking man who grew up in Chicago slums. He describes how he hit the bottle after he left the hospital.

"I drank to pass out. It was the only way I could get any sleep. I did that for a year, a fifth of booze every night. Finally I saw what I was doing: feeling sorry for myself. I'd wake up with the same pain I had before, plus a hangover. I quit drinking and joined AA and went into business. I've been dry for eighteen years."

Fred, in his way, is as tough and determined as Sam, but he is not going to waste his life pursuing "relief." His drive is focused on living as normal a life as possible.

"I'll tell you why I'm here. My family doc heard about this place and thought I should come here because you have some new treatments or something."

Fred leans over and puts his hands on my desk, wincing as he does so. "Listen, Doc, I hope I'm not being too crude, but I don't want to waste your time and mine, so if you can't help my case just tell me, and we'll call it quits, with no hard feelings."

He straightens up, slowly and stiffly. "I'm not going to take that much time away from my family, or from my business either."

The difference between Sam and Fred is important. Both are brave and tough. But Sam is on his way to becoming a "professional pain patient," disrupting his entire life as he embarks on a career of finding a nonexistent "cure." And Fred is using his toughness to fight invalidism, to keep what is precious to him; and he clearly begrudges every moment away from his usual life.

Clearly, if the pain is not severe, and if it is diagnosed as due to a common problem, such as back strain or tension headache or degenerative ("wear-and-tear") arthritis, then the most appropriate action is to follow the doctor's instructions and get on with the business of living. It is really not worthwhile to pursue endless further diagnoses. The remedies for these conditions, such as physical-therapy exercises and biofeedback for muscle-relaxation training, are simple and effective, and there is no need to seek a more exotic cure.

If no diagnosis has been made and you do not know what the problem is, then it is reasonable to get some answers. Or if there is a diagnosis but the treatment does not bring the pain under sufficient control to enable you to function effectively, then it is reasonable to ask for more adequate pain control.

The family physician may be very competent and a nice person who makes you feel comfortable, but such a generalist usually calls in specialists to help diagnose and manage unusual or difficult pain problems. You can expect to be referred to a rheumatologist if your joint pains are thought to be due to rheumatoid (inflammatory) arthritis, to an orthopedist or neurosurgeon for a spine problem, to a neurologist for chronic headaches or nerve damage, etc.

If you have seen such a specialist, and have been told what the problem is and that nothing further can be done to eliminate the cause of the pain, then you can feel fairly certain that you have taken reasonable steps. If there is any doubt, then a second opinion from another specialist can be obtained. If the diagnosis is confirmed—then no more shopping! You must face the fact that you may have pain for the rest of your life.

As we described in an earlier chapter, pain is not always a "warning signal" that something bad is happening; chronic pain is usually a "false alarm" which signals that damage has already occurred, as in a sunburn. The problem is usually not one of finding the cause; that is usually known. And it is not one of finding a cure; that usually does not exist. Rather, the problem is one of accepting the fact that the pain is going to be there indefinitely and that it is going to be necessary to learn how to live well despite the pain.

But even if there is usually no way to eliminate chronic pain completely, there are safe ways of reducing it significantly, or at least "taking the edge off" the pain. And, as this book illustrates, there are techniques for coping with the pain successfully. But it all begins with this attitude of accepting the fact of having the pain—not chasing after unreal diagnoses or impossible cures.

This acceptance is probably the most difficult step of all, but the most important. We have a natural, built-in reflex to avoid or escape pain, and our bodies seem to cry out that we do something—anything—to get rid of the pain. But after you have taken reasonable steps to determine if it is possible, you must be prepared to accept the verdict, "You'll have to learn to live with it." Once you accept the fact that the pain is here to stay, then your self-image changes, and you find that you can turn your attention to how you are going to manage the other aspects of your life.

Jim, an ex-Marine who was shot up in Vietnam, kept trying to convince surgeons that he could not function as long as he had pain. He wanted them to do some kind of surgery, any kind, that would eliminate the pain. Jim had been very physical all his life and could not imagine making a living in a way that did not involve hard labor.

One day, however, Jim decided he was not going to be able to get rid of his pain, and then his whole attitude changed, and his pain became easier to control. He took his hobby, raising exotic birds, and developed it into a small but profitable business.

"I feel the most important thing," Jim says, "is for the person who has pain to convince himself that he will have it the rest of his life and not try to fool himself."

Setting Goals

Once you have decided to accept your pain as a part of daily life, the next question to be answered is, "How do I want to live? What do I want to do that is realistically possible for me?"

By goals we do not mean something impossible like "getting rid of the pain," or vague and general, such as "keeping busy." We are referring to very specific achievements or activities, such as "getting a job as a bookkeeper," "working in the garden four hours each day," "taking the class in ceramics at adult evening school," etc.

In general, we need goals in three areas of our lives (this applies to almost everyone but especially to those in pain): in the area of work, or money-making activities; in the area of recreation or hobbies, or "fun" activities; and in the area of interaction with family, friends and others, or social activities.

Goals related to work are very important. I have known many persons whose pain prevented them from working at their former trade, such as carpentry, plumbing, electrical work, waiting on tables, etc. These people collected disability pensions and sat around doing little but complaining of their pain and their small income. It never seemed to enter their heads that if they couldn't work at their old trade, they could learn a new one. If they were asked what they did, they would say, "Well, I *used* to be a carpenter," or, "I'm a plumber, but I'm disabled now," etc.

This is a very negative identity to have. The homemaker who cannot take care of the home and the bricklayer who cannot do his job begin to have very low opinions of themselves. They feel useless and not needed. They do not really have a reason for getting up in the morning. They lie around, get fat, feel sorry for themselves, and all this makes their pain seem that much worse.

Ethel is 55 years old, divorced for many years and badly crippled with arthritis. Her children are grown, and although they live nearby, they are involved with their own families and only visit occasionally, although they telephone frequently. Ethel lives alone, but she is very happy.

"I'm a nut about gardening. I work in my garden about four or five hours a day. I can't stand or walk, so I had raised beds built and I kind of sit and drag myself along, and I can do everything I want to do. I don't know what I'd do if I couldn't take care of my plants."

It is very important for people in pain to have a work goal for several reasons: it may provide additional income; it gives them pride in accomplishment and in being able to overcome a handicap; it keeps them busy and less likely to get in poor mental and physical condition; and it keeps their minds off the pain so it is not noticed as much.

The homemaker who cannot do the usual chores may go into business, such as running a telephone answering service, and pay for someone to clean the house. The carpenter may become a locksmith, the electrician may do small appliance repairs, etc. It is always possible to do something different and worthwhile. If necessary, it is possible to contact your local government's vocational rehabilitation counselor. This trained professional can arrange to give you aptitude and interest tests, to have your strengths and weaknesses evaluated, and can help arrange for training in a new field.

Similar thinking can be applied to what you do for fun. Many persons can no longer bowl or play tennis or golf because of a bad back, cannot do needlework because of arthritis, etc. But those persons may learn to do artwork, such as pottery, printing, photography, or develop skills, such as archery, swimming, chess (even playing by mail!), etc.

There are scores of activities to choose from, and being involved in one or more is important. It gives you something to look forward to each day, a reason for getting up with pleasure and anticipation because you are looking forward to spending time doing something enjoyable. And time spent in enjoyable activity is "time out" from pain—the pain may still be there, but when you are absorbed in something else, it is not noticed as much, or doesn't seem to bother as much.

The third area in which goals are important is in improving your social life. Almost always, constant pain makes people irritable. Whether living with your family or living alone, you will probably have noticed a tendency to withdraw, to have less to do with others, not only because "they get on my nerves," but because of feeling ashamed of feeling snappish and grumpy, of being so cross with those you care about, for silly reasons or even for no reason at all.

As the old saying goes, "Everybody needs somebody," and it is not good to withdraw. The goal should be to increase and improve social relationships. It is possible to visit someone for coffee for a half-hour or so each day, or to have someone over. It is possible to call someone on the telephone just to chat or gossip or to keep up the old relationship.

It is important for you to realize that you *matter* to others, whether you think so or not, and whether you are in pain or not. It is no good to say, "They have their own lives," or, "They have troubles of their own, they don't want to hear about mine." The fact is, *you* are a part of their lives. And while they do have troubles of their own, they won't mind hearing about yours once in a while if you don't make a habit of it, and if you'll also listen to theirs.

But you don't have to talk about your troubles only. You can discuss politics, the problems with young people nowadays, how things were when you were growing up, etc. The point is that it is comforting to share other people's company, and just as when working or enjoying a hobby, the time you spend socializing is time you are distracted from your pain.

You will need to set your own specific goals in each of the three areas—work, recreation, and social activities. You need to have these goals as reasons for overcoming your pain. Everything else in this book is about *how* to cope with the pain. Your specific goals are the reasons *why*.

Using Anger

Although not all patients admit it, anger helped them start on the road to recovery, and anger helps to keep them going when they have rough spells. How? They angrily refuse to be kept down.

Anger is not bad when it is used in this way. It is not directed unreasonably at a person. It is directed at pain as a handicap and the frustration it causes. Used in this way, anger is a motivating force that can help you live the life you want to live, despite being in pain.

Here are three examples of patients who become angry and used that anger to overcome the effects their pain had on them.

Steve

A burly ex–Green Beret from New York, he had his lifetime career in the Marines cut short by mortar fire just two years before he would have been eligible for retirement.

"When I was first hurt, I used to get all this sympathy and pity, you know? The nurses and volunteers, how they'd look at you, you could tell what they were thinking. 'Oh, this *poor* man. What a *shame!*' Man, I used to eat it up. I really enjoyed feeling sorry for myself, saying, 'Yeah, I've really been shafted.'

"Then I got tired of the whole thing. It wasn't getting me nowhere, you know? I got so mad I almost hit those damn ladies when they came around. I checked out of that hospital and got a job as a karate instructor and started going to school at night."

Those "damn ladies" didn't realize it, but their "sympathy and pity" were so irritating after a while that they had the effect of angering Steve, and he directed his anger in a very constructive way.

Lyle

A navy pilot in World War II and a successful salesman afterward, he developed peripheral vascular disease which resulted in the amputation of one leg and left him with little use of the other. For nine years he had severe phantom pain (pain in the absent leg). For five of those years he did nothing but watch TV and visit doctors. Then, he writes,

"One morning I was sitting there [in the pain ward] staring out the window and thinking that old cliché, 'Why me?' You hit me right between the eyes with 'Lyle, you're a coward; you think this is all b.s., don't you?' Well, that did it! I got angry as hell and vowed to myself I'd show you and every bastard alive that old Lyle was still the best damn fighter that lived—not in the air anymore, because pain is the enemy. So I started. . . ."

Lyle, at age 57, became able to do fifty sit-ups and fifty push-ups every morning, and bench-pressed 350 pounds. Though confined to a wheelchair, he kept up the housework for his working wife, repaired and refinished their furniture and wrote the war history of his aircraft carrier. He clearly relates the start of his rehabilitation to a moment of anger.

Marcia

A 47-year-old housewife, who was on a vacation trip with her husband when their private plane crashed, Marcia has been paralyzed from the waist down and in pain for eight years now. But she keeps on doing all the things she used to do—housework, music, etc.—only slower, from her wheelchair. She writes,

"I believe I have an angry attitude. I am highly incensed that I must live like this. I don't blame anyone in particular, but I refuse to take the attitude that 'what will be, will be.' I resent this having happened to me, and I refuse to roll over and die."

Marcia has accepted the *fact* that she is paralyzed and will probably always have shooting pains in her useless legs, but she does not accept it as "right," nor does she let it stop her from living the life she wants. The worse the pain gets, the angrier she gets at it and the more determined she becomes.

"When the pain is bad," she writes, "I rise above it. It's a mental thing. The higher the pain goes, the higher my mind goes to surmount it."

Not only does the anger serve a useful purpose in helping motivate persons to start taking steps to do something with their lives; it helps them in their day-to-day progress. Those with chronic pain cannot afford to be passive and expect others to make them better. All that pain experts can do is point the way—explain what needs to be done and how to accomplish it. It is necessary for each one who has pain to take responsibility for his or her own progress, and anger at pain can help to fuel this responsibility.

It is understandable that hurting all the time can make you hesitant to begin to be active, so that gradually you adopt the behaviors of an invalid. We have the idea that if activity makes pain worse, some harm or damage must occur. This is sometimes reinforced by doctors who say, "If it hurts, don't do it." But this is rarely the case with chronic pain. "Hurting" does not mean "harming." And to resume normal living may require some more pain. It is anger at the pain that gives us the determination to start taking the necessary steps—and to keep taking them—to live the life we want to live despite the pain.

Having Faith

We have described how it is important to accept the fact of your pain, to set specific goals for living a satisfying life and to get angry at the pain, when necessary, to help motivate you to accomplish your goals.

But many patients find it essential also to have a religious faith. They view their pain as a message from God. It gives their lives a new meaning. They have to think through all the things they have taken for granted. Because chronic pain makes you think.

When you hurt all the time, it is natural to wish you were dead. You wonder if you can go on. You lie awake at three in the morning and wonder why you should continue living and suffering. Wouldn't others be better off if you were dead?

Answers come: I can go on, if I have faith; there must be a reason for this; no, they wouldn't be better off without me—my time will come later anyway. You begin to think about how we are supposed to live and what is really important in life. Your religion becomes even more important, not only for putting things in proper perspective, but for the comfort of such rituals as prayer, religious services, meetings of fellowship groups, etc.

Some patients have no religion and learn how to cope with pain without any religious participation. I have not been able to notice any outward difference in the success with which those with religious involvement live their lives as compared to those without religious participation. But I have the feeling that those with religion have an extra source of comfort and satisfaction, and a different perspective that is very important to them. They find that their faith gives them strength. There must be an inner difference, then.

In this chapter we have considered the attitudes necessary to start learning how to live with pain. Just feeling sorry for yourself doesn't accomplish very much—it is an understandable feeling and a natural one, but it doesn't get you very far. The right attitude of acceptance, constructive use of anger, having specific goals and faith prepare you to use specific techniques. All that has been covered in this book so far is an orientation. Now we come to the methods themselves.

4.
Strategies and Techniques for Pain Control

Generally speaking, there are two major approaches to pain control: that which alters the functioning of the body in some way and that which teaches mental control of the pain. Until about thirty years ago, physicians could only attempt to cut nerve pathways and prescribe narcotics, as they had done for hundreds of years. When this proved inadequate, they referred patients to psychiatrists or to ministers.

As we described earlier, traditional surgical attempts to alleviate chronic pain are disappointing. Narcotics usually result in many complications. And the role for psychiatrists and ministers is not usually one that benefits those with chronic pain. Fortunately, there have been many advances in the past 30 years—more than in the entire preceding 300 years—and far more varieties of help are available to control pain than were previously imagined. New techniques are appearing continually, so you and your family have every reason to remain hopeful that still others will become available that will be helpful.

In this chapter we will present an overview of pain-control techniques and describe their advantages and disadvantages. Then, in subsequent chapters, we will give more details about the specific techniques which you can use to help with the pain. Because many people have some magical hope that surgery can provide a cure, we will start with an overview of this approach.

Surgery

In Chapter 2, we indicated some of the general anatomical realities that make it very difficult if not impossible to eliminate chronic pain, but in this section we need to consider the surgical approach as a technique.

It should be obvious that there are many painful medical conditions that can be corrected surgically. Gall bladder disease, for example, or a herniated disk, or degenerative disease of a joint. If a person has pain due to disease of this sort (and there are other examples as well), and the underlying problem can be corrected, then of course this should be done.

But this is not really surgical treatment of pain; rather it is surgical treatment of one or another disease that has pain as one of its symptoms. There are many such conditions, ranging from appendicitis to tumors compressing nerves, and for each condition there are several medical and surgical approaches to be considered. In such situations, pain is really a side issue.

When a patient has a terminal disease, and pain is a serious problem which cannot be controlled adequately with analgesics or other alternatives, then a neurosurgical attempt at pain relief often brings very satisfactory results. Unlike the previous situation, in which surgery is used to correct a defect or remedy a problem, here the attempt is not to treat the condition but only to eliminate the pain.

Often the terminal disease is widespread cancer; especially

when the disease has spread to or involves the bones, the pain may be difficult to control with analgesics or radiation. In such instances, the neurosurgeon may offer the patient the option of cutting major pathways in the spinal cord (cordotomy), or possibly destroying a major nerve center like the pituitary gland (hypophysectomy). Depending on the specific condition and the location of the pain, other procedures may be considered.

The relief that cordotomies and hypophysectomies bring is usually immediate and dramatic. The patient is often able to discontinue analgesics altogether and remain clearheaded for the remaining several weeks or few months of life.

Why cannot this approach be applied to those whose pain is chronic but who are not near death? There are several reasons. First, such major surgery has a number of side effects. Some serious weakness of the legs and arms may occur with cordotomies, or lack of full awareness of where the limbs are. For a patient confined to bed, this is not important, but for others it may impair good mobility. Also, there may develop some problems with bladder or bowel control. Hypophysectomies change body chemistry dramatically, and although some replacement of chemicals is possible, in the long run it may be difficult to compensate.

But most important, the pain relief tends to become less effective with time. Some patients begin to notice a return of pain in a few months; many more within a year. Often the pain is markedly worse, with the addition of a state called hyperpathia—a marked sensitivity to normal stimulation, with an explosive pain response. It is not certain how the pain returns, and with it the additional unpleasant qualities, but recently evidence has been found for previously unsuspected sprouting of nerve fibers in the central nervous system: they apparently begin to regenerate after being cut.

So there is a role for surgery in correcting underlying problems and in alleviating terminal pain, but is there any similar role for this approach in chronic-pain states, in which pain itself is the problem? Yes, there are several kinds of pain states that can be alleviated by surgical treatment. Trigeminal neuralgia and causalgia are two painful conditions that have a surgical remedy.

Trigeminal neuralgia is pain in one of the branches of the trigeminal nerve. It is felt as intense spasms of pain in the face or head, which can be triggered by the slightest touch, by chewing or talking—even by a light breeze. It is thought that the pain is caused by the pulsing of a small artery in the brain as it lies against the nerve. There are at least three operations that work very well to eliminate this pain, if it cannot be controlled by medication. Although the operations are not without risks, the success rates are high and the results very gratifying.

Albert is a 64-year-old retired electrician whose haggard expression reveals his suffering. Periodically the right side of his face twitches, and he cries out in pain. He has intermittent electric-shock sensations, which occur about two or three times an hour. The pains can be triggered by talking, chewing, brushing his teeth or shaving. He has trigeminal neuralgia, an irritation of the cranial nerves supplying the face.

A neurologist has given Albert several kinds of anticonvulsant medications, which usually help this problem, but they have not worked. They only seem to make him groggy and uncoordinated, and he has fallen twice. It has been suggested that he have surgery, but this frightens him, and he has come for another opinion.

We discuss the three kinds of surgery that are possible: injecting an oily substance, glycerol, to desensitize the nerve center; making a radio-frequency lesion in the trigeminal nerve center; and open brain surgery to see if a blood vessel, whose pulsations may be causing the pain, is lying on the nerve.

Albert thinks that the glycerol injection doesn't sound too frightening. He makes an appointment with one of the neurosurgeons to get more details about the procedure and then elects to go ahead. When I see him again, it is a week following the surgery, and he is smiling broadly.

"See," he says, "I can talk and even touch my face. The pain is gone. I was a little numb there for two days, but that's gone now too."

I think Albert is probably still smiling.

Causalgia is a burning pain that is usually the result of an injury, such as a sudden blow or wound, that partially damages some sympathetic nerves. The nerves that regulate blood vessels seem to be overactive, causing the blood supply to that part of the body (usually arm or leg) to be greatly diminished. There is then an inadequate supply of oxygen and other nutrients to the tissues, and atrophy can occur. If the condition can be caught before serious changes occur, either repeated nerve blocks or cutting the sympathetic nerve fibers (sympathectomy) can alleviate the problem.

For the vast majority of chronic-pain problems, however, such as low back pain, joint pains, headache, muscle pains, etc., there is no neurosurgical procedure that is helpful. Some years ago, there was a great deal of interest in implanting electrical stimulators on the spine. This seemed to offer dramatic relief for some cases of intractable back pain. But the long-term success rate was poor, and now the procedure is done in only a few centers on an experimental basis. Similarly, there is some experimental implantation of electrodes in the brain for pain control, but this also cannot be considered a standard treatment as yet.

In addition to cutting nerve pathways or making lesions in nerve centers or implanting electrical stimulators, neurosurgeons have implanted small pumps and reservoirs to drip analgesics like morphine directly onto the spinal cord. The idea is that, because the analgesic can be used in very small amounts and lower concentrations, less tolerance to the drug develops. The technique is used primarily in terminal patients, however, and despite the theory, it has been found that the drug is taken up into the brain and drug tolerance develops anyway.

Nerve Blocks

Anyone who has been to the dentist knows that injecting a small amount of anesthetic around a nerve can make that part of the face and mouth temporarily numb. This type of temporary deadening of an area is called a local or regional anesthetic block. It is anesthetic rather than analgesic because it blocks not only pain sensations but all other sensations as well. The region involved feels dead or wooden or like some other inanimate object.

Can such temporary blocks help chronic pain? In some cases, such as causalgia, if the nerves are blocked repeatedly early in the course of the disease, it may completely reverse the problem. But in the majority of pain states the temporary regional blocks provide only temporary relief.

Such regional blocks, however, can be of considerable diagnostic help. By blocking one or another nerve pathway and observing the effects, it is sometimes possible to determine just where the problem is and, in some instances, to eliminate it. For example, chronic groin pain may be due to a number of causes, and the injury signal may be carried along the ilioinguinal or genitofemoral nerves. If blocking one of them relieves the pain temporarily, then a surgeon can explore that nerve and, perhaps, free it from adhesion or whatever else is causing the pain.

Similarly, differential spinal blocks are used to determine

whether sympathetic or sensory nerves are involved in a pain problem. Different concentrations of anesthetic are used, and depending on the result, the anesthesiologist can determine which part of the nervous system is involved. This can sometimes lead to a surgical procedure, such as a sympathectomy, which can resolve the pain problem.

If a temporary block can relieve the pain temporarily, could the block be repeated and made permanent so the relief would be lasting? There are many problems with this. The nerve must be killed, essentially, and the poison used to do this is alcohol or phenol. These toxic substances may spread and destroy much of the tissue surrounding the nerve, causing much pain and scarring and permanent damage. And the nerve itself may not be permanently destroyed but only partly so, and regrow, with additional pain symptoms developing just as in some surgical attempts to cut the nerve.

There are some instances in which such a "permanent" block can be very helpful. Most notable is the abdominal pain due to pancreatitis, whether resulting from inflammatory disease or cancer of the pancreas. For this condition, a temporary block of the nerve center supplying the pancreas, the celiac ganglion, may be found to provide temporary relief. In such a case the ganglion can be injected with alcohol to give very long-lasting relief, usually on the order of several months or more.

But most pain states cannot be treated this way. First, no one would want to risk damaging healthy tissue. Second, most would not want a leg or arm (let's say) numb and useless. And finally, the long-lasting relief is rarely permanent, endures usually only a matter of months, and repeated blocks are less and less successful.

Electrical Nerve Stimulation

The use of electricity for pain control has a very long history. The ancients used electrical fish. Aristotle, Pliny and Plutarch wrote of the numbing effects, and Scribonius described the technique used for treatment of the pain of gout and of headache.

Electrotherapy became more predictable and convenient with the development of electrostatic devices such as the Leyden jar. There were almost immediate reports of their use in pain relief. With the development of batteries, reports of electrical analgesia for surgical procedures also appeared. The technique waxed and waned in popularity and respectability in the eighteenth and nineteenth centuries, and electroanalgesia has apparently been "rediscovered" numerous times. We sometimes flatter ourselves that it is in our time that electrical techniques of pain control were developed and the ancient Chinese technique of acupuncture "discovered," but both methods were used fairly widely in Europe and the United States in the 1800s!

Both electrical stimulation and acupuncture appear to involve the same mechanisms of analgesia. There is now good research evidence, showing that stimulation directly inhibits spinal-cord spinothalamic tract cells from firing in response to incoming injury signals; their threshold for transmitting these signals toward the brain is raised considerably. In addition there appears to be an activation of brain stem descending inhibitory systems, which also raises the thresholds of these cells, and which involves such chemicals as enkephalin and serotonin as part of the gate control process.

When the first reports of acupuncture and electrical stimulation reappeared in this country in the early 1970s, there was considerable skepticism about their having real effects. Many persons suggested the analgesia was due to "suggestion" and would not work if the patient did not believe in it. There are now hundreds of controlled research studies which show that the mechanisms involved are physiological and "belief" has little to do with it. In research with animals, which have no reason to "believe" anything one way or another, electrical stimulation reliably raises pain thresholds. It is interesting that today Chinese and Japanese acupuncturists use electrical pulses in their needles for an enhanced analgesic effect. But there are also studies which show that vigorous vibration can produce the same benefits as electrical stimulation. Whether by use of needles or electricity or vibration, the analgesic effect is the same once the peripheral nerves are stimulated.

The majority of studies show that when the peripheral nerves are stimulated vigorously, there is a maximum analgesic benefit reached in about twenty minutes in that region of the body being treated. When the stimulation is stopped, the analgesic effect wears off slowly, in about an hour or two.

There is an exceptionally convenient form of electrical analgesia that has been available (on medical prescription) since the early 1970s. Known now as TENS (transcutaneous electrical nerve stimulation), it is a small battery-powered pulsing stimulator that can deliver current to several pairs of electrodes. The device is convenient enough to be worn under the clothing, and stimulation can be either periodic when the need is felt, or continuous. A range of pulse rates, strengths and widths is available so that various kinds of stimulation are possible for the different kinds and locations of pain. Patients can experiment to learn what works best for their particular pain problem.

We have already mentioned that neurosurgical techniques for implanting stimulating electrodes around nerves, on the spine and in the brain, though initially showing much promise for certain very desperate causes of pain, are disappointing as to long-term results.

TENS seems to have a variable long-term success rate, depending on the type of pain problem it is used for and the setting in which it is used. When pain is widespread in the body, TENS is less effective. When the pain is localized in a small area, TENS is much more effective. When TENS is used alone for pain control, about 50 percent of all pain patients receive significant relief with it, but this success rate declines to about 30–35 percent after one year. When TENS is used as a part of a comprehensive pain management program, including the use of all the techniques described in this book, then the success rate improves about 65–70 percent initially and about 50 percent at one-year follow-up.

Marjorie is a very young-looking 73-year-old woman. Two years ago she had a bout of shingles, a painful eruption of blisters around her left lower chest and flank. After several weeks this eruption, caused by the herpes zoster (chickenpox) virus, ended, but the nerve damage it caused persisted, with continued burning and jabbing pain and hypersensitivity of the skin. This is post-herpetic neuralgia.

A variety of medications had been tried, with little success. Marjorie complains of her life being so miserable now that she doesn't want to go on living. She and her husband had been enjoying their retirement, living in a trailer park, socializing with other couples. Now she doesn't go visiting, nor does she have visitors over. She just sits and watches television and goes for short walks. She is so miserable with "this damn pain" that she is nearly past the point of desperation.

We place a set of TENS electrodes in the mirror image of her painful area on the opposite side of her body, on the right. The left side is too sensitive. For three days she receives intense electrical stimulation for thirty minutes four times daily. On the fourth day the electrodes are finally placed on the left side, near the painful area, and the stimulation continues.

"I don't know if it's all in my imagination," Marjorie says, "but the pain isn't as bad."

"It may be just wishful thinking," I warn her. "Don't jump to conclusions. We need you to be a careful observer of the effects of this stimulation."

"If it's wishful thinking, I'll take it. I'm more comfortable."

The trial period is over now. Marjorie only needs to use TENS twice a day to maintain its effects, and she and her husband have resumed their social activities.

There are few problems connected with TENS. Addiction does not occur, as with narcotics. Patients with cardiac pacemakers should not use it, although this can be evaluated by a cardiologist, as new pacemakers are shielded against such electrical stimulation. Skin irritation is sometimes a problem but disappears when stimulation is stopped. In general, TENS is a quite safe and moderately effective method of reducing pain. But it clearly works best when it is just one of a variety of techniques, physical and mental, used for pain control.

Chemical Pain Control
Apparently since the earliest times, humans have used chemicals for a variety of purposes. Virtually all peoples have used alcohol in one form or another, as well as a variety of plants for medicinal purposes. The plants used for analgesia form the basis of the analgesics we use even today. Although we now make synthetic analgesics and no longer need to rely on plants, the basic kinds of analgesics are essentially the same as they have been for a long time.

There are dozens of brands of analgesics, but the confusion about them can be lessened considerably by understanding that there are just two basic types: those that work "out there" in the body, where the injury signals originate; and those that work in the central nervous system—brain and spinal cord—where the injury signals are processed.

There are just three nonprescription analgesics that work to inhibit the start of injury signals where the damage has occurred. Aspirin is the best known of these, acetaminophen (e.g., Tylenol) and ibuprofen (e.g., Nuprin) are the other two that are available over the counter in the U.S. All of them seem to have the effect of raising the thresholds of free nerve endings so that they do not as readily signal that injury has occurred. In addition, aspirin and ibuprofen (but not acetaminophen) have anti-inflammatory effects and block certain of the chemical changes which occur in tissues that have been injured and, in this way, also serve to reduce pain.

Many persons with severe long-standing pain dismiss these nonprescription analgesics as having no effect on their pain, but this is usually not completely accurate. Often they wait until the pain is almost unbearable, then take several tablets without noticing any benefit and so think they are of no value. This is not the proper way to use analgesics in chronic pain. We describe how to use them in Chapter 8.

The other major class of analgesics, which works directly on the central nervous system, is that of the opiate drugs, the narcotics. There are a number of these, ranging from codeine to morphine, but all work on the same principle. They all inhibit cell activity by occupying the morphine (mu) receptors on cell membranes. Thus they slow, or completely block, the transmission of injury signals to the thalamus and to the parts of the brain's cortex that help to localize and interpret the pain.

But pain transmission is not the only function of the body that reacts to these opiates. Patients who complain of constipation, inability to ejaculate, clouded thinking, trouble coughing when necessary and slowed breathing are noticing the complications and side effects of using narcotic analgesics. Some patients have said that these drugs do not really block pain but only "fool their mind" into thinking there is no pain. This is not really correct, because it can be shown that these analgesics really do reduce the number of injury signals going to the brain. But because some pain may still be felt and thinking is less clear, it is understandable that this interpretation may occur.

Since the systematic use of anesthesia and opiates began in the last century, surgery and childbirth and the treatment of trauma have become less hellish and more humane. After surgery or trauma, we are fortunate indeed to have these analgesics available. So too in the treatment of painful terminal illnesses. But there are serious problems with these narcotics when used for chronic pain—problems of tolerance, dependence and conditioned pain responses. We will describe these in Chapter 8.

Since all current narcotic analgesics have these drawbacks—supressing the cough reflex, depressing respiration, constipation, etc.—and since it has now been found that there are at least three other kinds of opiate receptors in the nervous system besides the mu receptor, there is much research going on now to develop new types of analgesics that will be as effective in pain control but without such drawbacks. This is very promising, but it will be some time before such compounds, when discovered, will be available.

Aside from the analgesics themselves, there are other kinds of medications that are very helpful in controlling pain. These are the so-called "psychotropic" medications, which are used for controlling emotional disorders but are also useful in raising pain tolerance levels.

In acute pain—for example, when minor surgical procedures are to be done, or postoperatively, or following injury—anxiety is usually present. Anxiety tends to make pain worse, or less tolerable. Antianxiety medications are quite effective in reducing pain intensity and make it possible to give less narcotic without reducing the analgesia produced. Patients feel more relaxed, less apprehensive, and so do not escalate their pain unnecessarily. And since less narcotic is needed, fewer narcotic side effects occur.

In chronic pain, however, depression often develops, as we described earlier. In such instances, antianxiety medications can make the depression worse. Antidepressant medications are very helpful, though. They improve sleep, appetite and energy levels, and seem to improve the patient's pain tolerance. A number of studies even show that antidepressant medications have a direct analgesic effect in addition to their antidepressant action. They are thus very helpful in managing chronic pain.

Until three years ago, Raymond was a comptroller in a major high-tech company, one which he had helped to form with some venture capital he and his partners had obtained. The job was stressful and the hours long, and three years ago, at age 53, Raymond had a stroke. He lost the feeling and use of his left side, though his mind remained clear.

In physical rehabilitation, Raymond began to recover some use of his body and was able to walk again. Then, two years ago, he began to experience the pain. At first it was mild, but it has gradually worsened. It is a deep, burning aching in his left side. Even though he is numb, the pain is present. With this pain he has become depressed. He dwells on his forced retirement and feeling of uselessness. His wife is becoming more worried about him. She reports that he has stopped doing his exercises and just sits, staring at the wall.

This kind of pain is called "thalamic pain," because it is due to degeneration of cells in certain inhibitory areas of the thalamus. And depression following strokes is not at all uncommon. When there is such severe and long-standing pain, the usual poststroke depression is much worse.

Raymond was started on an antidepressant, amitriptyline (e.g., Elavil), to be taken each night, and in two weeks he began expressing an interest in doing his exercises again. In two more weeks he felt that his pain was no longer a serious problem, and his wife reported him to be more like his usual self.

Now Raymond is thinking of doing some volunteer work. He has very good business experience and is planning to do volunteer counseling to small businesses unable to hire consultants. He continues to keep up with his daily exercise routine and says that, although he still has pain, it is now only a mild aching, which he can live with.

Antianxiety and antidepressant drugs all require medical prescriptions, and for patients with certain medical conditions these medications may be somewhat risky. But generally speaking they are safe and, when used for a short period of time, can help the patient to acquire control of the pain problem.

There are other kinds of medications, too, that are helpful in certain specific pain conditions. For example, there are those which partially inhibit the sympathetic nervous system and thus alleviate the pain associated with injury to sympathetic nerves. There are medications primarily used for epilepsy but which are helpful in controlling neuralgias as well. The point of mentioning these is to show that there are a variety of chemical agents available by prescription, in addition to opiate analgesics, that can be of significant value in controlling and, at times, eliminating pain.

Body Treatments

Aside from electrical and chemical manipulations, there are a wide variety of body stimulation and manipulation techniques that can reduce pain. Physical therapists use heat packs, ice packs, massage, ultrasound, etc., to relax muscles and reduce inflammation and pain. Chiropractors manipulate the spine, and a variety of different massage techniques—often named after the founder of one or another theory or "school"—poke and prod and stretch various parts of the body.

Some of these types of body stimulation use strange explanations about "lines of energy," follow patterns of "pressure points" and "energy centers" on the body surfaces, and often combine their technique with recommendations for a certain kind of diet and food supplements. Most of this is probably harmless.

When the pain problem is primarily due to strain of the muscles and ligaments, such massage and stimulation techniques can result in a good and lasting reduction of pain, especially if some muscle contractions have followed the stretch injury. But when pain is due to almost any other cause, the vigorous stimulation will provide only a temporary reduction of the pain, just as does TENS, vibration or acupuncture. This is called a "counter-stimulation effect" and is probably due to the same mechanism involved in TENS, namely the temporary raising of the threshold of spinal-cord cells to incoming injury signals.

Most patients with chronic pain from any cause appear to develop a muscle pain component as well. This may be due to "favoring" a sore leg, or to sitting or lying down too much and becoming deconditioned, or it may be due to muscle contractions and spasms. When such muscle pain occurs—and it is a common problem in chronic low back pain and in tension headache—it may respond temporarily to such measures as heat and massage, but usually pain recurs, and for the same reasons.

What is effective in such cases of chronic pain is a physical rehabilitation and conditioning program. It consists of a gradual and progressive conditioning of the entire body and not only improves the immediate muscle pain component, but also prevents reinjury. It makes it possible for those with chronic pain to function much more effectively. It is a major component of most pain treatment programs, and generally patients consider it one of the most important parts of their treatment. Physical therapists also like this conditioning and rehabilitation better than manipulation techniques because they get satisfaction from seeing the patients improve and remain better, rather than come back time after time for more heat, ice and massage.

We will discuss the techniques of physical rehabilitation further in Chapter 5. However, it is important to note here that physical conditioning is not meant primarily to control pain, but to improve functioning despite pain. It may incidentally reduce the muscle component of pain, and by means of daily exercise pain tolerance may be improved, but these are simply side benefits rather than the main purpose.

Psychological Approaches

Physical conditioning and psychological training are probably the two main pillars of any pain treatment program. The tasks of the psychological part are:

- to determine how much of your pain and disability may be due to psychological factors, such as depression, family problems, financial or job difficulties, etc.;
- to determine what factors in your environment might be (unconsciously) contributing to excessive pain and disability;
- to determine whether you are thinking about the pain, its sensation and its meaning, in such a way as to make the pain worse than it need be;

- to work with you and your family to reduce and eliminate all excessive pain and disability, in order to enable you to resume normal functioning.

There are two major ways of thinking about the pain problem from a psychological perspective. One is behavioral and is concerned with habits—the way your behavior is reinforced by things that happen. For example, if a child with pain gets much-needed attention from neglectful parents, then there is a greater likelihood that the child will show pain when he or she next has a powerful need for the parents' attention. The idea here is that the pain behavior has been rewarded by attention. Sometimes the parents may ignore or even punish the child if they suspect the child to be faking in order to get attention. The child may then learn to have real "accidents" with painful injuries in order to get the needed attention. Such attention is needed because, in the absence of a normal loving relationship, attention is, at least, a substitute for love.

Adults also can have their pain behavior rewarded—by getting out of unpleasant or stressful work situations or a difficult relationship, by receiving narcotics or by whatever else the person may need. It might seem as though pain is a very high price to pay for such rewards (reinforcers), but for some it is worth it. It is not that these reinforcers *cause* the pain; they do not. Rather, they make the pain more disabling and longer lasting than need be. For one patient, for example, whose relationship is on the rocks and whose partner shows concern about the pain, it is a lot easier to bear the physical pain than the emotional "pain" of seeing the relationship end if the patient gets well. The pain persists because it is reinforced by the attention of the partner who might otherwise leave.

The other major psychological view of the pain problem is from a cognitive (mental) perspective. This refers to the way you think about your pain. For example, if you think that pain is *always* a "warning signal," no matter how many months or years it has been present, then you will continually be in a state of alarm about the pain, forever consulting doctors and not getting on with the business of living.

Cognitive processes consist in part of the things we tell ourselves about a situation or condition. With chronic pain, it would consist in large measure of the "silent conversation" inside your head about what the pain means or represents. You might tell yourself that if the pain has persisted for such a long time, then it must represent a malignant disease that is too subtle for the doctors to discover yet, and by the time they do find out it will be too late. Or maybe they already know but are keeping the truth from you to spare your feelings, because it is hopeless. In either case it must be that the underlying cause of the pain is something deadly. There is no point to going on or hoping for any relief, because things can only get worse.

This kind of thinking, of course, soon leads to invalidism and a chronic bedfast state, with a progressive worsening of your condition. As you become sicker, your fears are confirmed in a self-fulfilling prophecy. There is thus little hope for rehabilitation and learning to live a good life despite chronic pain until your erroneous thinking can be corrected. We all have interpretations of our symptoms; if our ideas are inaccurate they can get in the way of our getting better, and cognitive therapy may be necessary before any other treatment can be effective. There is little point in showing back exercises to someone who believes that the back pain is a sign of progressive paralysis, for example.

Both of these psychological treatments—changing the habits or behavior patterns and changing the incorrect or harmful ways of thinking about the pain—are usually essential to dealing with pain successfully. In most pain treatment programs, a combined approach is used and is referred to as "cognitive-behavioral therapy" for pain. It takes place in individual, group and family counseling sessions, and proceeds along with the physical-therapy program, trials of TENS, training in relaxation techniques, etc. We describe the cognitive-behavioral approaches in greater detail in Chapter 6.

5.
Physical Conditioning

Just as having the right attitudes makes all the difference in psychological control of pain, so physical conditioning is the most important factor in enabling you to make your body do the things you want. In nearly every case of chronic pain, the patient has an *excess* of pain and disability—more pain and handicap than is necessary—due to physical deconditioning as much as to depression and other psychological factors.

The reason that most pain patients have more pain than they need to have is because of the effects that pain has on them, as we described previously. Because of the pain, there is a tendency to be inactive. And because of inactivity there is boredom and frustration. And because of boredom and frustration there is nervous snacking and a gradual weight gain.

The problem with being so deconditioned is that it causes muscles to become strained and weak and painful. This can greatly worsen a chronic-pain problem, such as low back pain due to chronic muscle and ligament strain. And it can add to the total amount of pain from any other problem. The inactive person tends to have less tolerance for pain in any case, as compared with those who exercise regularly. It is thought that exercise may stimulate the production of those brain chemicals—endorphins, enkephalins and serotonin—which raise pain tolerance.

For these reasons it is very important to get into the best physical condition possible within the limits of your disability and to work every day at keeping fit. In purely practical terms, there is a very big difference in the ability to cope with pain between those who get in good physical condition and those who do not. Pain specialists see this every day. So do pain patients notice the improvement, comparing themselves before and after treatment. When I sent follow-up questionnaires to patients one year after they had completed a pain treatment program and asked them what had been the most useful part of the program, they overwhelmingly considered the physical-therapy exercises to be the most important and helpful part of the treatment they received.

Evaluation
The great majority of patients with chronic pain cannot be damaged by activity and exercise despite their feeling that the pain gets worse when they are physically active. But this does not mean that you should just plunge in and start a vigorous calisthenics program. That could lead to an injury. Each case is different, and no two cases of back pain or nerve damage or joint pain are exactly alike. Each person needs to have a set of exercises developed for his or her own particular condition.

There is only one sensible way of doing this, and that is under the direction and supervision of a registered physical therapist. This trained professional is given a prescription for your treatment by your physician so that due allowance can be made for your actual physical condition.

Frances is 34 years old and has had two back surgeries. The first was done for a herniated disk, which occurred when she lifted one of the small handicapped children in her class. The second was done to remove a disk fragment that was left behind (or recurred) after the first surgery. Her back and leg pain are the same as before. She has remained incapacitated and bedfast because her doctor has said to her, "If it hurts, don't do it."

Evaluation now fails to show any need for further surgery or any need to restrict activities. It is thought that her pain is due to scar tissue and physical deconditioning. The situation is explained to Frances, and she is eager to begin a rehabilitation program. She is tested in the physical-therapy department and, as might be expected after spending weeks in bed, she is found to be very weak. The occupational therapist finds that Frances is very limited in most of the activities of daily living.

A program is developed for her, and Frances performs a full set of exercises under supervision twice a day. It is necessary for the therapists to take her husband aside and give him special instructions. He brings Frances to the clinic each day because she cannot drive yet. He is very overprotective. When the therapist has her start a certain exercise, he says, "You can't do that, you'd better be careful," etc. Without intending it, he has been contributing to her excessive disability.

Within six weeks Frances is functioning quite normally. There is nothing she did before that she cannot do now. She is obviously pleased. And her husband, who has been doing the exercises with her, is proud of her as well. They take long walks in the evening after dinner and are now planning camping trips with their children.

You and your doctor should understand that the physical therapy you need is not one of hot packs, massage and ultrasound, as might be appropriate for an acute strain or injury.

That sort of treatment is pleasant and comforting, but accomplishes nothing as far as long-term treatment of chronic pain is concerned. Since the physical therapist must follow the doctor's prescription, you will want to discuss with your doctor just what treatment he or she is ordering from the physical therapist.

If your doctor agrees, the prescription or order should request evaluation and rehabilitation for your chronic-pain problem, using behavioral techniques (see below) as part of a general conditioning program that includes aerobics conditioning and special attention to the painful area (such as neck, back, leg, etc.).

The reason for mentioning the behavioral techniques is that just showing you some exercises to do at home accomplishes very little. The behavioral techniques, as part of the rehabilitation program, will be described later in this chapter. We are talking here about a really serious rehabilitation program. You need to become as fit and completely able to function well as possible. This program by itself will probably not help your pain, or help it only a little, but it will certainly enable you to achieve the specific goals you set for yourself in the areas of work, recreation and social activities. And the behavioral techniques used as part of the physical-therapy program are designed to help maximize your likelihood of succeeding in the program and minimize your chance of failure.

In some rehabilitation centers, your evaluation will be done by a physiatrist, a physician (M.D.) who specializes in physical medicine and rehabilitation. This physiatrist will also supervise the theapists' treatment of you. In other centers the physical therapists do the evaluation and treatment on their own, under the general supervision of a medical director. In pain treatment programs also, physical therapists who specialize in treating patients with chronic-pain problems will do their own evaluation and carry out your treatment under the general supervision of a medical director.

Your evaluation, whether by a physiatrist or physical therapist, consists of testing you in a number of ways to see how weak or strong you are in each muscle group, how stiff or flexible, sore or tender your muscles are. He or she will examine your ranges of motion, the way you sit and stand and walk, how well you can perform the activities of daily living, what your endurance is and your cardiovascular functioning, etc. In such an examination, which may take an hour or two for two or three consecutive days, it will quickly become apparent just what your areas of weakness are and also just how many and what kinds of exercise you need to become functional again.

The physical therapist will then have you try to do each kind of exercise you need, doing as many repetitions of each one as you can. This, like the rest of the evaluation, is likely to leave you feeling pretty sore for a few days, but it is important so that the therapist can know at just what level of each exercise you need to start your program.

Conditioning Principles

Your therapist will set reasonable and practical goals for each of your exercises—and you may have a dozen or more exercises given you for your total conditioning program. For example, suppose you have weak abdominal muscles—you should be able to do twenty bent-knee sit-ups or leg lifts and can only do six. Or, you may be so out of shape that you can only walk briskly or ride a stationary bike for five minutes, although you should be able to do so for thirty minutes. A plan must be made to bring you up to your exercise goal safely over a period of several weeks.

Now, here is where the first behavioral principle comes into effect. Instead of doing as many repetitions of each exercise as you can each time and hoping you improve each day, as is customary, in this technique you begin working on the pre-scribed exercises at a level just one-third of your present tolerance and do them twice daily. For example, if you could only do six sit-ups or leg lifts when you were tested, your therapist will have you start by doing just two at first, morning and afternoon, along with your other exercises.

What is "behavioral" about this? And why use this system? It is designed so that you will be likely to succeed and unlikely to fail. For example, if you were able to do six leg lifts, you should have no problem doing two of them twice a day. And after two or three days, you should be able to do three without any trouble. And in two or three more days, you should have no problem doing four leg lifts twice a day. And so on. Within a short time you will be doing six of them, with far less trouble than you had when you were tested, and then you'll go on until you reach your goal of twenty. At that point your therapist will have you cut back to just one exercise period a day to maintain your fitness at that level.

The advantage of this method is that, by starting at one-third of your tolerance, you should have no problem with the exercise and no increase in pain with it. Therefore you do not associate a worsening of your pain with the activity, and you can also feel assured of success at each small increase in exercise along the way. Furthermore, by exercising twice daily until you reach your goal, you improve your ability far more than if you did this only once a day, so that every two or three days you can make a small increase in the number of repetitions and do so easily. And you will do this for each of the dozen or so exercises. The aerobics—whether biking, walking, swimming, rowing, etc.—you'll increase just one minute every few days, for the same reason, and find yourself able to pass your initial maximum easily in just a few weeks.

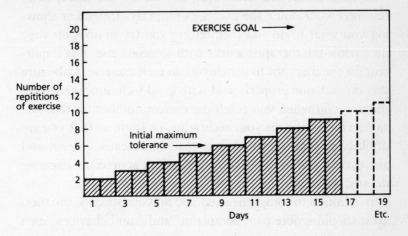

Fig. 1: Exercise graph. A graph like this is made for each exercise. Progress in increasing the number of repetitions of each one is followed and charted systematically. Exercises are done twice daily until the goal is reached, then maintained at that level once a day.

The second behavioral technique is the use of a graph for charting your progress on each exercise. This seemingly simple device allows you to keep careful track of just how many times you are supposed to be doing each exercise and to mark your progress on each one twice daily. This helps you to progress smoothly; to avoid mistakes, such as overdoing, which might lead to more pain; and to keep track of your progress. Patients also find these graphs to be a kind of reward, a source of considerable satisfaction, as they see themselves go past their initial maximum level of repetitions easily and move ahead toward their exercise goals. The graphs are all collected in a binder, like a booklet, and you'll mark each exercise as you do it, twice daily, so you can follow your progress day by day—and show it to others as well.

A third behavioral technique is used by the therapist to reinforce your doing the exercises properly. Instead of showing you what to do and then letting you try to do it on your own while the therapist works with someone else, it is important for the therapist to watch you do each exercise, make sure you do each one properly and with good technique, and compliment you when you reach the correct number for that session. This reinforces your technique, or form, so that you are unlikely to pick up bad habits that might cause injury, and also gives a pat on the back, which we all appreciate when we do any task well.

In addition to complimenting you on your success, the therapist should ignore pain complaints and pain behaviors, such as grimacing, moaning, limping, etc., because all such behaviors have to stop if you are going to function normally. You have the opportunity to show all those kinds of pain behaviors while you are being evaluated and tested on each exercise. It is what helps to determine what kind of exercises you need, what your initial tolerance is for each exercise and therefore at what level you should start your exercise program. Since you'll be starting at only one-third of what you can do, there really should be no problem once you begin the exercises, and all such pain behaviors and complaining are unnecessary and serve no purpose except to proclaim to the world that you are suffering. Therefore, to help you overcome this bad habit— which you must drop if you are going to reenter the world of normally functioning human beings—the therapist ignores these pain complaints and behaviors and pays attention instead just to your healthy behaviors and conversation.

Since you have been hurting and out of commission for so long, you have probably picked up more of these habits common to people who are sick or disabled—talking about your symptoms and how bad you feel, how many pills you've taken and doctors you've seen, etc. It is all about the things that preoccupy you. But it is awful stuff to have to listen to and drives other people away. Keeping that frown and pained expression on your face, sighing or grunting with effort, limping or clutching your back are similarly unacceptable. None of this does any good. It doesn't help your pain. It is merely an expression of how bad you feel and a way of declaring to the world that you are a disabled and suffering pain patient.

These kinds of behaviors are appropriate for acute pain. They help to communicate your needs and get you the help you require. But when pain continues for months and years, perhaps indefinitely, such pain behaviors and complaints no longer serve any purpose. No further help can be forthcoming except what you can do for yourself. Neither family nor friends nor medical persons can do any more to eliminate your pain. You have told them all about it, your case has been studied, you know that nothing more can be done except to get back to functioning normally again despite the pain—so you must stop all these behaviors. That is why the therapist has to ignore them, to act as though you are not doing them so that you'll stop. Obviously, you've kept them up because they've brought you some attention. The therapist—and others in the program as well—expect that you'll stop all that carrying on when you stop getting attention for it. Then you'll be able to move on to more normal behaviors.

For this reason as well, family members are brought into the treatment program, partly to teach them about this technique so that they do not continue to reinforce your invalidism. Usually, families have tended to cater to patients because they think they should and feel guilty if they don't. They must learn that such attention to pain behaviors is appropriate for acute pain but useless if the pain is chronic and does not represent an emergency. In fact, such family reinforcement of pain behaviors can actually sabotage a patient's efforts at rehabilitation. We will discuss the role of the family further in a later chapter.

Finally, it should be obvious to you that if you continue to think about your pain, talk about it and act it out with your behaviors, then you are "living" your pain. You are never apart from it. Yet you need as much time apart from your pain as you can possibly get. It is a basic psychological principle that, just as thoughts can influence feelings and behavior, so can behavior influence thoughts and feelings. If you shape your speech and actions and thoughts to normal, healthy, everyday standards, you will find yourself gradually less involved in your pain and less aware of it. The pain may still be there and may not change, but you will force it from your consciousness as you become more and more involved in such nonpain behaviors as exercising and taking steps toward satisfying your work, recreation and social goals.

So do not think your therapist is being coldhearted and indifferent for not giving you a lot of attention and sympathy. He or she is giving you what you need—rehabilitation. After all, you got all that sympathy and attention before, and it didn't make you any better. Rehabilitation will help you get better—not necessarily in changing your pain, but in enabling you to function better and lead a more satisfying life. This business of ignoring your pain behaviors after the evaluation is almost always explained to you during the orientation phase in pain programs and by your physical therapist if you are in a therapy center elsewhere. It is part of helping you learn to start being tough with yourself, because you are not going to achieve your goals unless you force yourself to make slow and steady progress toward normal functioning.

In order to make progress, you will have to keep to a rigid schedule of twice-daily exercising despite ups and downs in your pain level. It will do you no good to think about the exercises but not do them, or do them in a sloppy way, or skip occasional exercise sessions. No one can force you to get better, and no one else is fooled or harmed by your not adhering to the schedule that has been worked out for you. If you don't follow through, others will draw the obvious conclusions about your motivation.

If you follow your exercise graphs, you'll probably reach most of the goal levels in about six to eight weeks, although it won't be the same for each exercise. Your therapist may well have adjusted the rate of change of some of your exercises to meet your condition—slowing down some you were having trouble with, speeding up others that were easier for you. But eventually you'll reach the goals set for you and then cut back to exercising just once a day to maintain your fitness level. You will need to be tough with yourself at this point, too, sticking to your program indefinitely, no matter what, so that you don't get out of shape and functioning poorly again.

Activities of Daily Living

The purpose of all the stretching and strengthening exercises is to improve the conditioning of your body so that you can do anything necessary to achieve the work, recreation and social goals that are going to bring you some satisfaction (and take your mind off your pain). The exercise goals are not ends in themselves, but means to the end of achieving your life goals.

(However, I have heard of a patient with back problems in another pain clinic who went far beyond these basic exercises to more strengthening exercises with weights. Then he went further still, becoming a body builder. His pain is as severe as ever, but he is working now as a fitness instructor. For this patient, the exercising became an end in itself, which he adapted to meet his career goal.)

Many times, in addition to a general conditioning program, a person may need some special training in order to be able to perform certain necessary tasks. Bending, lifting and carrying heavy objects (such as bags of groceries), reaching objects high on a shelf or below a counter are all necessary to normal household functioning. Or you may need to be able to stand in lines, or sit in a classroom or an office, or climb stairs.

These kinds of things are called ADLs, or activities of daily living. If your exercises do not improve your ability to deal with such tasks, your therapist, or an occupational therapist, will develop graphs similar to your exercise graphs for these specific activities, starting you at a level well below your initial maximal tolerance and then helping you increase the amount you do every few days until you achieve your goal for each activity. This gradual and progressive increase each day will enable you to accomplish the tasks you need to do, with no increase in pain and without doing yourself any harm.

Kevin is a big, husky 36-year-old disabled police officer. He was involved in a fight with a prisoner who was attempting an escape while being transferred from jail to prison. Kevin was injured in the back and chest and has had recurrent muscle spasms that take away his breath. He was placed on restricted duty for six months, during which time he just did paperwork, and he received physical therapy. When he was unable to return to full duty, he was given medical leave, and if unable to resume his duties in another six months, he was to be placed on disability.

Kevin tried more physical therapy and then worked with an exercise physiologist at a sports medicine center. Nothing seemed to help—whenever he did the exercises, the spasms would start. He became discouraged. The six months passed, and he was discharged on disability status.

After evaluation to make sure there are no other significant medical or surgical or psychological problems, Kevin has been started on the behavioral physical-therapy program. He started at just one-fourth the number of repetitions of his initial maximal tolerance, is exercising twice daily and increasing by just one repetition every three or four days. On this schedule, he is not having spasms, although he has been in the program for several weeks now. He is optimistic about being able to work again, but does not plan on returning to the police force. He is bitter about having had to retain a lawyer to sue the city in order to get the disability income he was supposed to have received regularly. Because of his unfortunate experiences with the city, Kevin has required some psychological counseling as well as physical re-habilitation. But he is very satisfied in having regained the physical abilities which are so important to him.

Aerobics
It should be obvious that, as no two individuals have the same pain problem, each person will need a different set of exercises, or need to start at a different level and to increase repetitions of each exercise at a different rate. A proper exercise program is tailored to meet the condition and goals of each person. The general goal is one of improving your ability to function normally by helping to develop your strength and flexibility and endurance. Your endurance is aided not only by the gradual increase in the number of repetitions of each exercise, but also by the improvement in your cardiopulmonary (heart and lung) functioning, which comes with your aerobic exercise.

By aerobics is meant the kind of exercise that increases your intake and use of oxygen. It need not be just the aerobic dance kind of exercise, although that could be one type you'd enjoy. Brisk walking, riding a stationary bike, jogging, using a rowing machine, swimming laps, etc., are all aerobic if done properly. To get the full benefit, you have to do the exercise fast enough to get your pulse up to your target heart rate. Of course, you'll need proper medical authorization for this, especially if you have heart or blood-pressure problems.

The target heart rate is calculated by subtracting your age from the number 220 and then taking 70 percent of the resulting number. For example, if you are 47 years old:

$$
\begin{array}{r}
220 \\
-47 \\
\hline
173 \times 70\% = 121
\end{array}
$$

You should be tested to see how long you can walk fast, let's say, and keep your pulse rate at 121 beats per minute. If you can do this for, say, eight minutes before you get too winded or your legs get too tired, then your therapist will make a walking (or biking, or whatever you choose) graph for you, starting at two or three minutes of brisk walking twice each day, with an increase of one minute every two or three days until you reach a goal of thirty minutes of good aerobic activity at your target heart rate. There will always be a period of two or three minutes, slow warm-up before the exercise and slow cool down afterward.

You may wonder what this kind of exercise has to do with your pain problem. There are two reasons for including it as part of your rehabilitation. One is that there is some preliminary research which suggests that aerobic exercise of this kind stimulates an increase of certain chemicals in the brain, such as serotonin and possibly enkephalin or endorphin, that improve our pain tolerance. So it makes it easier for us to bear our pain. One or more of these chemicals may also combat the depression associated with chronic pain. There is some evidence that aerobic activity of this sort is as effective for this type of depression as antidepressant medication.

The second reason is that aerobic exercise seems to be a good way of discharging muscle tension and the feeling of emotional tenseness that accompanies any kind of stress, including pain. The irritability that pain patients report is a reflection of this kind of stress reaction, this feeling of inner tightness and tenseness. Almost all patients notice an improvement in this condition when they do their aerobics and report that they do feel better afterward. Of course, they are also improving their capacity to work and their endurance, so their goals are more easily achieved.

Carole is a 52-year-old woman who has worked as a secretary since graduating from high school. She has never done any exercising and has been experiencing more and more headaches and back pains. Evaluation has revealed that she has some scoliosis (curvature of the spine), tension headaches and physical deconditioning.

Since starting her behavioral rehabilitation program, Carole has been feeling remarkably well. Not only is she free of headaches and back pains, but she is "turned on" by her brisk walking and stationary bike aerobics. She does one in the morning and the other in the evening, before and after work. Carole is one of those fortunate people who feel "high" after a good aerobic workout. She is so pleased with this program that she is planning to join a health club when she finishes. She is working with the physical therapist to develop additional exercises she can do at the club.

* * *

Your choice of aerobic exercise depends upon your preference. You should choose the kind of activity that you *can* do and will stay with. For most patients with joint or spine problems or headache, bouncing or jarring exercises should be avoided. This would rule out jogging, bouncing on a trampoline or in aerobic dances, etc. The smoother activities such as stationary biking or brisk walking or working out on a rowing machine or swimming laps would be fine, and your choice depends on what is available to you and your preference. You can work this out with your therapist. Some patients like variety and so alternate biking and walking, or do an outdoor exercise in good weather and an indoor one when the weather is bad. Choose what you like, but be faithful about it.

We have gone into some detail about the physical-conditioning program so that you understand what is done and the reasons for it. We cannot give more specific details of just what exercises you need because each case is different and requires a unique program. You need professional supervision. But if you think you can make up your own exercise program, be sure to get your doctor's approval first, to make sure you do yourself no harm. Then follow the principles we have outlined, of starting slowly and increasing gradually to a level appropriate to your age and ability. And remember: exercises are merely a means to an end. They are designed to help you achieve your work and recreation and social goals. If you don't have such goals and don't pursue them, getting in good physical condition won't make your life much more satisfying to you.

Avoid Stimulants

We should not end a chapter on physical conditioning without pointing out that it is important to avoid those substances which increase muscle tension and blood pressure. Caffeine and nicotine do this. All caffeine—in coffee, tea, chocolate, colas and some nonprescription analgesics—has this effect, and so does tobacco. The result is a worsening of the kind of stress reaction caused by the original pain itself, the mimicking of the fight-or-flight pattern, which prepares the body for the emergency signaled by the pain. This pattern of responses is all very well for true emergencies, but is harmful in long-term, chronic-pain states. If you smoke and drink coffee, you may think it is relaxing to do so, but that is only because you are calming your withdrawal symptoms when your body "needs" the coffee and cigarettes. Actually, these substances are increasing your irritability, tension, nervousness and restlessness, and making your muscles tighter and more likely to cramp or go into spasm.

For the sake of your pain, as well as your general health, you must give up these substances altogether. If you cannot do it yourself, discuss techniques for doing so with the psychologist you see to learn the psychological techniques we describe in the next chapter.

6.
Psychological Techniques for Coping with Pain

Many persons with chronic pain are nervous about psychological strategies and techniques for coping with pain. Even when their pain is due to known nerve damage or adhesions or a similar obvious cause, these persons believe that if you can make your pain less severe by psychological (mental) methods, then that means the pain was "all in the head" (psychologically caused) in the first place. This is a false belief.

In fact, some of the best mental control of pain comes in such settings as burn units, where patients are so badly burned they are too ill to be given full doses of narcotics, yet need to be bathed and have dressings changed twice daily. Hypnosis, relaxation skills, visual imagery and similar mental techniques have been very helpful in controlling such pain. Similarly, cancer pain can be controlled by these methods and often has been. Surely, no one would suggest that the pains of burns and cancer are "all in the head"—they are in the brain, of course, because that is where we become aware of them, but they are not psychologically caused.

Surprisingly enough, it is psychologically caused pain that is likely not to respond to psychological treatments. In fact, it doesn't respond well to any pain treatment—not medication, not surgery, nor anything else like that. This is because the patient needs the pain for some psychological reason. The only treatment that can help is psychotherapy to uncover that reason and to help the patient find better solutions. We will discuss this further in Chapter 7.

Most persons with chronic pain, although they may be nervous about psychological pain-control methods, are nevertheless willing to try them because they are eager to look into any *safe* way of reducing their pain. But they usually admit to being very skeptical, even doubtful. It is hard for people who are hurting all the time, who have tried to fight their pain, tried to ignore it, tried to distract themselves from it, etc., to believe that some mental tricks can block out pain. You probably have the same reaction. You have probably tried every trick you can think of, and nothing works very well, and that is why you are reading this book now—to learn if there is something else that can help you, because so far nothing has. And so it's nearly impossible for you to imagine that different ways of thinking can reduce pain, or even eliminate it at times. After all, if your pain can awaken you from a sound sleep, what can you possibly do while you're awake to block out the pain?

You may also think that, since you are so skeptical, these techniques cannot work for you, because you have to believe in them for them to work. That is not true, either. In fact, you should remain skeptical, because that will make you a less biased observer. You will be able to report more accurately just exactly what you notice when you try these kinds of mental control of your pain. You will be able to discover what makes your pain worse, what makes it better and what has no effect. By becoming an accurate observer of how thoughts and feelings influence your pain, you will have taken the first step toward acquiring the skills of mental pain control.

Even patients who are afraid others will suspect that the pain is "all in the head" are quick to admit that their pain usually gets worse when they are emotionally upset—when they have a quarrel, for example, or feel pressures of deadlines, or there are financial or family problems, or similar kinds of stress. It is certainly a well-reported fact that such feelings as anxiety or anger can make pain worse. Thoughts and feelings actually can make pain better as well as worse, and in this chapter we will describe how.

However, you must understand that just reading this chapter will not give you any skills for controlling your pain. You must actually practice the techniques, apply them regularly and get good at them. It is very like learning a foreign language. This chapter could describe what you need to do to learn one, but you wouldn't learn the language by only reading this chapter. You'd have to practice and drill. What this chapter does do is describe different kinds of mental pain-control techniques, giving some examples. In reading about them, you may very well remain highly doubtful that they can help, because they seem very simple. However, they can and do help thousands of pain patients—but you have to actually practice them to get any benefit. These mental skills are every bit as useful and important as are the physical conditioning exercises.

Attitudes and Attention

When we described attitudes toward pain in an earlier chapter, we were really describing ways of thinking about ourselves and about our pain. These attitudes are based on commonsense ideas so obvious that we don't usually think of them as "psychological" or "mental," although they are. The ways in which we think about ourselves and our pain strongly influence our ability to cope with the pain. If we fail to make goals for ourselves, we will have little motivation for overcoming the terrible effects pain has. If we are pessimistic and negative, thinking of ourselves as chronic invalids, we surrender to an unsatisfying life of excessive pain. This is one example of how the way we think can have an effect on the pain we experience.

We also have mentioned several times how being absorbed in a task can provide "time out" from pain—the pain may still be there, but you are not noticing it while you are absorbed in something else. This also is a "mental method" that we will be describing further, because it is a skill that can be developed and used more efficiently than you may realize. Like having positive attitudes, being distracted, absorbed or involved is so obvious and such a commonsense approach to pain control that we tend to forget that it is a psychological technique, and also that it works.

In the last chapter, we mentioned that one of the effects of not reinforcing pain behaviors is to help shape you toward more normal functioning. As you give up groaning or limping, or making pained facial expressions or complaints of pain, you begin to start feeling more normal. As you come closer and closer to your exercise goals and can sit and stand and walk for longer and longer periods without worsening your pain, you become less able to think of yourself as a disabled or handicapped person and feel better because your actual behavior is not consistent with your self-image of being disabled. This is an example of how behavior influences thinking and feeling.

And as we described with respect to attitudes, the opposite also is true. If we think of ourselves as hopeless invalids because of our pain, we stay home and do very little and feel terrible about ourselves and our lives. But if we change our attitudes, and also our other ways of thinking, we can reduce or control our pain and start doing more satisfying things and feeling better as well. This also is an obvious and simple idea, yet everyday experience tells us it is true, and it is important to keep it in mind as you read about the various techniques.

Let's try a small experiment. While you are sitting or lying down and reading this, notice the sensations that are coming from your thighs and buttocks. You can feel the pressure of the surface you are on as it presses the clothes against your skin. You can feel the warmth and the wrinkles in the material on your skin. They are real physical sensations, not uncomfortable, but just there. They have been there all this time, but until your attention was called to them you did not notice them, because you were thinking about what you were reading. Your attention is like a radio tuner. Radio signals from many stations are in the air all the time, but you hear only the one you are tuned to. The same is true of your body's sensations. The pressure on the skin of your thighs and buttocks was there all along, but your attention was not focused on it, so you did not notice it.

The same principle applies to your pain. Like another radio station, its signals can be there; but if you are not tuned to it, you need not notice it. Not noticing can be important and helpful to you. You can be so absorbed in something, so interested and involved in something you are doing, that you do not notice your pain. As soon as your attention is directed to it you feel it again, unchanged. It does not go away. But you tune out your pain the way you change the radio dial—you tune in on something else. What you pay attention to, what you focus on, is up to you. You can shift your attention to something outside yourself, or you can shift your thoughts to something in your imagination.

Negative Assumptions and Thoughts

If we have the assumption that pain is *always* a warning signal, then even unchanging chronic pain must be a sign to us that we are in danger, and we spend our time frantically searching for an explanation.

If we basically believe that pain is a sign that we are sick, then we give up dealing with everyday life and spend our time in bed or visiting doctors until we are well—even though we have had the same pain for many years and nothing else has developed.

If our assumption is that pain is a disability, then we surrender the possibility of being able to earn a living or being able to function very well at anything until the pain is removed.

These basic assumptions are not at all correct, but if we believe them, then they give rise to certain negative thoughts bound up with equally negative feelings. Because we tell ourselves continually every day that we are sick or disabled or have something wrong with us, we keep our mood down and our skies gray and become capable of little enjoyment. As a consequence, the negative thoughts gradually become self-fulfilling prophecies. As we go doctor-shopping and stock up on drugs, we feel less like our old selves. We do less, stay home more, act more like invalids, become deconditioned and feel more ill. This confirms our assumption that we are not well, so we do even less, take more drugs, etc., and feel still worse about ourselves.

All this only magnifies our pain because we dwell upon it as the source of our troubles, and the more attention we give our pain, the more we notice it, the bigger and more intense it looms in our minds. It occupies us, dominates our thinking and feeling, and so it comes to dominate us altogether. In this way the negative thoughts are much more serious and dangerous in the long run than most of us ever suspect.

Psychological Techniques for Coping with Pain · 101

Challenging False Assumptions

Before you can get very far with psychological techniques of pain control, you obviously need to identify your silent assumptions and self-defeating thoughts and change them. This is much easier if you are working with a psychologist who knows something about you and can ask the right kinds of questions to bring out your unspoken assumptions and thoughts. But you can do some of this yourself, if you are willing to ask yourself the hard questions and not evade the answers.

What do you think your pain means? What is causing it? Are you sick, or disabled? If so, is it because of the pain? Are your answers to these questions ones that you have made up and believe, or are they professional opinions?

It is considerably easier to change such ideas, and the negative thoughts and feelings which they generate, as you start on your physical rehabilitation and exercise program. As you begin to be more active, as you feel yourself become stronger and more able to do things, you start to challenge the negative basic assumptions. It is easier to see yourself making some progress in overcoming the pain handicap, and so you begin to question some of those incorrect ideas.

In the same way, you must start to catch yourself when you begin these negative conversations or upsetting automatic thoughts. It is helpful to write it down when you notice yourself thinking or saying such things as:

- This pain is terrible, I don't know how much longer I can take it.
- I can't do that because of this pain I'm in.
- Things are really bad, I'm going to have to see the doctor about this.
- I can't stop thinking about this pain; I feel like a hypochondriac.

*　　*　　*

What you want to do is to note when you get these thoughts, what the situation is, what things led you to think about the pain and your inability to cope with it. You need to see the relationships among the situation in which these thoughts occur, the things you say to yourself about it and how it makes you feel. When you begin to see and understand how your bad feelings arise not only from the pain itself but from the things you say to yourself about certain situations or events, then you will be able to stop negative thinking and start reacting in a more positive way.

You will be able to start substituting more positive and realistic statements that more accurately reflect the true situation, such as:

- I've had flare-ups in the pain before, and it settles down again; nothing to worry about.
- I'm going to hurt as much whether I do it or not, so I might as well do it.
- The docs don't have any answers for this; I'm just going to have to get going on my own.
- I've got better things to do than brood about this pain.

The more you change your way of thinking, the more you will find yourself interested in doing things differently. And this is why it is so useful to begin the physical (and behavioral) approach at the same time, because it gives you the constructive things to be doing and reason to believe that you are really going to be able to overcome the pain after all. So the physical rehabilitation and the psychological techniques reinforce each other and help you make more steady and certain progress toward your goals.

If you are in a pain program or treatment center, it is very likely that you will have the opportunity to participate in group sessions with other pain patients, during which you will discover a variety of ways in which people with pain have learned to talk themselves into excessive pain and disability and a "professional pain role." Under the guidance of the psychologist, you will have the opportunity to observe how certain events or situations lead to certain negative feelings and automatic thoughts that reinforce the pain and make it worse. Then you will practice using more realistic and positive approaches to such situations and events—things that come up at home, or when shopping, or at work—and perhaps even role-play or act out more positive ways of coping with these situations. By rehearsing them, you develop better strategies and skills for dealing with things that can occur in your life and for coping with pain.

Coping Techniques

In this section we will describe some specific ways in which you can manage your pain more successfully, but we should point out that some first steps for coping with pain have already been described and cannot be ignored, because what we will be describing next builds on them. These first steps are:

- setting specific goals and making plans regarding work or worklike activities, recreation or hobbies and social activities;
- beginning a behavioral physical-therapy conditioning program as described in the previous chapter;
- examining your basic assumptions about your pain, and your negative thoughts, and changing them, as described in the previous section.

Once you have taken these first steps, it will be much easier to apply the following techniques. But if you have only read the preceding material and not begun to do anything about taking steps, these techniques will probably not seem very promising and will not be easy to apply.

"Move Your Muscles, Change Your Thoughts"

This basic rule is a slogan of Recovery, Inc., a self-help group of former mental patients, and it is exceptionally useful for persons with chronic pain as well. From long experience with thousands of mental patients, Recovery, Inc., learned many years ago that when a person begins to feel bad, feels a depression or "spell" coming on, then it is very important for him or her to change what he or she is doing and thinking. The bad feeling or thoughts are very likely tied in some way to the specific situation that person is in at the time, what that person is doing or thinking. Therefore, to change the reaction, to prevent the bad feelings or thoughts from getting out of hand, it is essential at the first awareness of the reaction to "move your muscles, change your thoughts."

Many pain patients themselves have discovered this principle. For example, the great majority of those with severe chronic pain have trouble sleeping through the night because the pain awakens them and they have trouble getting comfortable enough to get back to sleep. Some just lie in bed, worrying about getting enough sleep, wondering what the pain means, what terrible disease it might represent, whether they have told the doctors everything or if they have missed reporting some important clue, fearing they will not be able to bear up under the pain any longer, etc. Such terrible thoughts run through their minds, making their pain escalate out of control.

But I know many other patients who simply get up and go to another room and go to work on a project, some handwork or artwork or shopwork or writing. They become absorbed in it, and when they feel themselves getting sleepy enough again, they go back to bed. They don't like being awakened by pain either, but when they are they react calmly and matter-of-factly, using the time for something they like that takes them away from escalating their pain. This is an excellent illustration that the principle of "move your muscles, change your thoughts" applies to pain as well as to emotional bad feelings.

Other patients I know have discovered that whenever they experience a flare-up of their pain and begin to have morbid thoughts about it, whether in the day or night, it is very helpful to go through their exercises an extra time (except for the aerobics). They feel it is like striking back at the pain, as well as helping their own rehab progress. Still other patients prefer to use their biofeedback tapes, going through the relaxation procedure to relax their muscles and calm their minds. (We will be describing this shortly.) This too is effective and follows the same principle of changing what you are doing and thinking in order to prevent the pain and your reactions to it from getting out of control.

Since you will have some specific conditioning exercises to do and will have started increasing your activities, the idea of "moving your muscles" should not be a difficult one to accept. You will also have planned some specific work and recreational activities that are realistic for you, so you should have some projects or activities around that you can involve yourself in. Thus we do not need to go into any further detail here about the kinds of things you can do to "move your muscles" to break the pain cycle. What we will need to do, however, is to specify some techniques for "changing your thoughts," because this seems kind of mysterious to many people. But you need to be able to "change your thoughts" too in order to overcome flare-ups of pain and the negative thinking and feeling which not only result from it but can contribute to it.

Hypnosis

Many people can go into a trance state and block out pain. A trance is a mental state in which you are awake and able to see and hear and often remember just what is going on, yet able to so focus your attention that you can change your usual way of thinking or feeling or remembering.

A normal example of this is your mental state just as you are drifting off to sleep or just awakening. For a few moments you are conscious, aware that you are awake, but not really aware of your body sensations nor your surroundings. You are not thinking any thoughts. You are simply aware, sort of like a mind floating in space, just noticing.

In hypnosis, these few moments can be extended to many minutes or even hours. In this time, suggestions given by the hypnotist, or by you yourself, if you are doing self-hypnosis, can be much more effective than if given in the waking state. If you are having leg pain, for example, you can imagine your leg going numb and the pain disappearing—and that is what you will feel. You can mentally soak a burning hand in ice water to relieve it.

Some very impressive results have been reported in thousands of cases using hypnosis alone for pain control, and still more are reported regularly in nearly every new issue of the scientific journals on hypnosis. Surgery, including amputations, using only hypnosis for anesthesia; changing dressings on hospitalized burn patients; control of migraine pains, etc., have all been reported repeatedly. Many films and videotapes of these procedures have been made, demonstrating quite vividly how effective hypnosis can be for pain control.

What is not much reported, however, is how many people try hypnosis and fail to get any benefit from it. Some with chronic pain notice much less pain while in the trance, but as soon as the trance is over the pain returns, unchanged. This seems to be the case for 20–25 percent of the general population. Only about 5–10 percent of the people who try it seem to be good enough at hypnosis to get some carry-over of pain relief when they are not in a trance state. More than 50 percent of the population report either no pain relief at all, or only a slight amount, which doesn't seem to help very much.

There seem to be two reasons for this. One is that individuals differ a great deal in their ability to go into a hypnotic trance and to develop such hypnotic skills as blocking out pain sensations. Some are very poor at it, others are quite remarkably good and still others have in-between degrees of ability. Practice seems to help a little, but not very much.

The other reason has to do with the skill of the hypnotist who teaches the patient self-hypnosis. The hypnotist may be excellent or poor or something in between. Being a good hypnotist seems to be a skill, just as being able to experience a trance is a skill. Training and practice seem to help the skills of the hypnotist somewhat more than they help the skills of one trying to experience a hypnotic trance, however. But it has become clear from a good deal of clinical research that, while some persons never acquire the ability to use hypnotic pain control effectively, no matter how much they practice and try to change the pain, others seem to develop this ability very quickly and easily, almost seeming to teach themselves.

Debbie is a 23-year-old receptionist who used to be a model until her accident. She put a chemical down her kitchen drain, which was clogged, not knowing her landlady had put another kind in the drain earlier. The chemical exploded, burning her chest badly. She tried to rinse herself off, but the water had been turned off.

In the burn unit of the hospital, where she spent several weeks, Debbie learned to put herself in a trance to tune out the pain when the dressings were changed twice daily. She became so good at this that she could do some startling things with self-hypnosis.

"I got bored with just lying there with nothing to do, no one to talk to. So when the nurse would come around to check my pulse and blood pressure, I'd trance myself out and pretend I was dead. I'd drop my pulse and blood pressure so far down that she'd call a code blue on me—thought I was dying. Everybody came running and stayed around a while, so I had company. I didn't do it all time though, just once in a while."

If you have a chronic-pain problem and would like to learn to control pain through self-hypnosis, this is very much worth trying. In fact, hypnosis may be the safest and simplest technique of pain control of all and should probably be the first one tried, rather than the last. Being able to control the pain with hypnosis does *not* mean the pain is caused mentally. In fact, as we have said, hypnosis works better on physical pain, because those with mentally caused pain usually have a psychological need for it and don't want to give it up (until their problem is solved).

So by all means ask your doctor for the name of a reputable professional who uses hypnosis in his or her practice. This should not be just someone who advertises or does hypnosis stage shows, but a physician (M.D.) or psychologist (Ph.D.) whose reputation is well known to your doctor. The local medical school, university hospital, or city (or county) medical or psychological societies are also sources of referrals to reputable professionals. And of course your local or regional pain treatment center may also teach hypnosis as a part of their program.

But you must remember several points before you start trying hypnosis. First, it will not be enough simply to try to block out pain with hypnosis and then continue living the same limited, disabled, unsatisfying life that you are living now. The hypnosis will not provide a miracle cure. It is only a technique, a tool, and controlling pain (eliminating it completely or just reducing its intensity) is just one step in getting your life on track again. You must specify clearly to yourself just what your goals are, what you want to control your pain *for*. You want to achieve some worklike activity, some recreational and some social goals. And whether or not hypnosis works for you, you must push on toward those goals, with both the physical conditioning and mental techniques.

The second point to remember before you try hypnosis is that the chances are it will probably only help somewhat—you may decrease the pain to some degree, perhaps just "take the edge off" your pain. Only a very small percentage of persons can block out pain sensations completely. So you must be realistic and not have such expectations of magic that you are bitterly disappointed if this method doesn't work for you. Give it a try by all means, have a half-dozen sessions with the physician or psychologist and practice the technique daily as you are instructed. If it is helpful, you will be very pleased and will not need to be reminded to keep using hypnosis. But if it is not helpful, do not give up on everything else.

The third point is that it has been found that there are other mental techniques for pain control that are good substitutes for hypnosis. They do not require an ability to go into a trance state and so can be used by everyone. Probably they work better for some people than for others, just as hypnosis does, but almost everyone can acquire some of these mental skills. We are going to describe these in the following sections of this chapter so you will know about them, but they really need to be taught in a training program. Most pain treatment centers include one or more of these methods in their programs.

*   *   *

Carl had been a heavy smoker. He knew all about the risks of cancer, but he always figured "by the time I get it, they'll have a cure." But his two packs per day caught up with him, and at the age of 57 he had cancer of the tongue and cheek. He needed surgery and then radiation treatments. By the time I saw him, two years later, Carl had a constant burning pain of the mouth, probably the effects of the radiation.

Although a serious-minded manager of a furniture store, Carl was willing to try anything that might help his pain. Analgesics were losing their effectiveness, and anyway he didn't like their side effects. He needed to suck on ice cubes several times a day in order to get a few moments of relief.

Carl proved to have an excellent ability at self-hypnosis and imagery. After training, he could just imagine himself sucking an ice cube and receive the same soothing benefits as when he was actually doing it. And since he could do this anytime he wished, without stopping whatever else he was doing, he could keep the pain under control.

Guided Imagery

Most of us use mental imagery throughout the day. It is like daydreaming. We imagine ourselves in certain situations, either reliving a recent event and changing it in our minds to make it come out better, or rehearsing a situation we are anticipating so we can prepare for any possible outcome. Or we may daydream about peaceful scenes, such as camping by a stream, fishing a quiet lake, lying totally relaxed on a beach, etc. Some of us have more vivid imaginations and can be so absorbed in such mental scenes that we can hear the sounds of the water, feel the warm sun, smell the fragrances and feel as though we are actually in the scene. Others experience these images less intensely, but nevertheless most of us daydream to some extent.

The average person can be trained to use imagery deliberately in this way. We have mentioned that when pain becomes more severe, along with the depressed feelings that accompany it, then it is important to change what you are doing and what you are thinking. It is for this reason that you can benefit from using mental imagery in a deliberate fashion—it is a way of changing your thinking to get you out of the bad state. You can get into a scene of your choice, preferably (though not necessarily) a relaxed and peaceful one, and live it so vividly that you leave the pain behind for a while.

The psychologist who trains you will probably ask you about some of your memorable pleasant experiences, some trips or vacations that make you feel good all over again when you recall them. Then you select one to become your favorite escape. If you have not had such an experience, the psychologist may suggest one to you. Then he or she will "talk you through" the experience. You will walk through the spring meadow (let's say), listening to the bird song and hearing the drowsy buzzing of the bees and croaking of the spring peepers. You see the rainbow colors of the spring blossoms against the pale green background of the meadow grass and breathe deeply of the delicate fragrances. The soft ground gives a light spring to your step, warm sun makes all your muscles relax and you feel the tensions draining out of your body. You walk slowly around the meadow, noticing the small rabbits scurrying into their little tunnels as you approach. And so on. The "trip" may take about twenty minutes or so.

As you see and hear and smell and feel this scene, engaging more and more of your senses, you become more and more absorbed in the imagery; you live it, and gradually you leave your present circumstances behind. Your pain and sadness recede into the background of your awareness and become less and less distressing. You are giving your mind and your emotions a much-needed rest. Most persons feel refreshed by this kind of experience. They feel calmer and more relaxed and peaceful, as though they had had a restful and refreshing nap. This technique is called guided imagery, because it is like a guided tour through a favorite daydream, not just a few brief scenes but a leisurely and totally involving stroll through a beautiful scene.

The psychologist will probably tape this scene for you so you can practice with it two or three times daily, and other scenes may be taped on other days so that you have a small library of these tapes to work with. You will be able to alternate the imagery so that it always seems fresh to you, and each scene has the power to make you feel restored and renewed. As you become more and more practiced in the technique you will be able to take these mental trips without the tapes, from memory, with the same benefit. Thus, when you need to "move your muscles, change your thoughts," you will be able to do so, and so get control of yourself and your situation again.

Many psychologists who use hypnosis claim that guided imagery is really hypnosis by another name. They say that, to the extent you become absorbed in the imagery (or any daydream, for that matter), to that extent you are in a trance. Others claim that imagery is similar but not the same, because special skills become apparent in a trance that are not seen in guided imagery. What's in a name? It really doesn't matter whether this technique is the same as hypnosis or only similar as long as it is helpful to you. It does appear, however, that guided imagery can be used by many who do not seem able to go into a deep hypnotic trance. At a guess, I suppose that some 70 percent of pain patients can used guided imagery well for pain control, compared with about 25 percent who get help from hypnosis. However, more and more hypnotists are using imagery techniques as well, to make hypnosis more effective for pain control, and the differences become blurred.

Another point to remember here is that many patients have different expectations for hypnosis and for imagery. There is a hope that hypnosis will cure pain as if by magic, and this is often fostered by foolish hypnotists who think that dogmatic statements promising relief of pain will produce good results. But this is bound to lead to much disappointment and poor results. Guided imagery is recognized as meant primarily to give a temporary "time out," and unreasonable expectations are not fostered; therefore, a higher success rate occurs. If patients only anticipated the same temporary relief from hypnosis that they do from guided imagery, perhaps with some slight carry-over afterward, there would probably be the same high rate of success for both techniques, with little disappointment.

Relaxation Techniques

Just as you "relax your mind" with hypnosis or guided imagery, it is important to relax your body as well. Pain causes a great deal of physical tension—muscles tighten, adding to the pain; blood pressure often increases as well; more and more energy is used, and you feel drained and exhausted. Most patients with chronic pain seem to have lost the ability to relax completely. It is as though the muscles develop a life of their own from the habit of tensing and bracing against the pain, and the ability to relax the muscles voluntarily seems to have disappeared. Even in sleep the patients clench their jaws, perhaps grind their teeth, tighten their fists and awaken feeling even less rested than when they went to bed. (Remember that nicotine and caffeine make this all much worse and should therefore be given up completely.)

Consequently, training in relaxation techniques can be very

helpful because it breaks the cycle of physical tension and stress in the same way that guided imagery breaks the cycle of emotional tension and stress. In some ways it is easier, though, because relaxation is usually not a new skill but something to be relearned. After all, most of us are not born being tense; rather, we develop tension as a reaction to some stress. So we simply need to learn how to let go of the tension and reacquire the ability to relax when we choose to do so. We need to learn also to catch ourselves starting to tighten up so that we don't let the tension escalate, but relax before it gets out of hand. And we also need to be able to relax as we function throughout the day, taking care of our daily business while remaining inwardly calm.

There are several methods for this relearning of relaxation skills, and they have a number of different names, but we will describe briefly just a few basic ones: breathing techniques, progressive muscle relaxation, autogenic training and biofeedback. These methods differ in *how* they get you to the point of deep relaxation, but the *goal* of all of them is the same: learning to relax quickly, easily and deeply and then to maintain an inner relaxed calm while you go on about your daily affairs.

Controlled breathing techniques.   One of the oldest and simplest relaxation techniques is that of controlled breathing. With this method you can slow your heart rate, lower your blood pressure and relax tense muscles within a short time. To begin, choose a time and place in which you are alone and undisturbed. No one should be at the door, the phone should be off the hook, TV and radio should be off, etc. Choose a spot in which you can lie or sit comfortably with spine straight (if lying, don't fall asleep). All this preparation is for the purpose of having nothing to distract you or make you uncomfortable for at least twenty minutes.

While sitting comfortably with spine straight, close your

eyes and relax all your muscles as best you can, thinking about each part of your body from the top of your head to the soles of your feet, relaxing each in turn and keeping relaxed.

Now concentrate on your breathing, breathing naturally through your nose, with your lips lightly closed, but jaw relaxed and teeth apart. Focus your attention on your breathing, and as you breathe out, say the word "calm" silently to yourself. Each time you exhale, say "calm" and feel the tensions drain away as you do so. When your mind wanders, as it always will, just be patient and focus your attention again and again on the feeling of your breath as you exhale and say "calm."

Keep this up for twenty minutes, checking the time occasionally, then open your eyes and sit quietly for a few minutes, then finally get up and continue your day's activities while you maintain the inner feeling of calm. Practice this twice a day, to get the most benefit from it. It breaks up the pressures of the day and enables you to feel calm, relaxed and restored. For most people it is best to have a regular routine, practicing this controlled breathing at the same time and place each day.

Progressive muscle relaxation. When muscle tension is a major problem, it is helpful to work directly on muscle relaxation. Again it is best to sit erect, but if this is too uncomfortable it is acceptable to lie flat or recline. Again choose a quiet place in which you will be undisturbed for at least twenty minutes.

Beginning with your feet, curl your toes and tighten them as much as you can, feeling all the muscles in the feet tense. Feel this tension for about ten seconds, then relax the feet completely, noticing how the toes uncurl and the muscles feel tired and heavy. Pay particular attention to the differences you notice when the muscles are tense and when they are relaxed. Now tighten the muscles of the legs, making them as stiff and rigid as possible and, holding that tension for at least ten seconds, notice how that feels. Now relax the legs, letting them go limp, and feel the difference.

In this way progress through alternate tensing and relaxing of the muscles of the buttocks, of the abdomen, of the back and neck, of the jaw, of the hands and arms. When you have tensed and relaxed each set of muscles of your body, remain still while you mentally check your muscles and experience them being very heavy and relaxed. Notice the feeling of deep muscle relaxation throughout your body.

Autogenic training. This technique, which originated in Germany, consists of repeating certain phrases to yourself as you focus on relaxing various parts of your body. As before, you need to have a quiet place in which you can be undisturbed for about twenty minutes and to sit or lie comfortably, spine straight.

Beginning with your feet, say to yourself, "My feet are heavy and warm, very heavy and warm." Repeat this several times, until you can actually *feel* them become heavy and warm. While you say this, picture your feet in warm water, or near a fireplace, gradually becoming warmer and heavier. Then do the same for your legs and each part of your body up to your scalp. By repeating this phrase to yourself and visualizing your body becoming heavy and warm in this way, you promote greater blood flow to the muscles and muscle relaxation, and you can feel as relaxed as if you had fallen asleep on a warm, sunny beach.

Of course, this use of relaxing phrases and visualization of the relaxation process can be combined with progressive muscle relaxation. First you tense and tighten muscle groups, then relax them. Then you repeat the appropriate phrase and picture each part of your body in turn being heavy and warm. By

Psychological Techniques for Coping with Pain · 117

first tensing the muscles, the subsequent relaxation is made more noticeable. Then repeating the phrase while visualizing and *feeling* the heaviness and warmth makes the relaxation still more complete. Once you have progressed slowly in this way throughout the entire length of your body, you should feel as limp as a cat asleep in the sun, totally loose and relaxed.

Biofeedback. Biofeedback requires equipment. It is a technique for measuring what is going on in your body and displaying it to you instantly as it occurs. Thus *biological* functions are *fed back* to you immediately so that you can modify them as you wish. For pain patients, the most useful functions to record and display are usually muscle tension and hand or foot temperature. This is because the usual stress reaction to pain includes an increase in the production of adrenaline, which causes muscles to tighten more easily and blood vessels in the hands and feet to constrict so that hands and feet become cold.

Many persons have been tense for so long that they actually do not relax when they think they are doing so. Even when they go to sleep at night and believe they "must be" relaxed, they are not, and recordings of muscle activity can show very high levels of tension. Such persons can practice controlled breathing and progressive muscle relaxation and autogenic phrases and still never actually relax because they seem to have forgotten how or no longer recognize what relaxation feels like. The clue that this is the case is that they do not feel any lessening of the pain with relaxation, nor do they feel refreshed or restored when they think they are relaxed.

In such cases, biofeedback is of invaluable help. You are hooked up to the equipment by a trained biofeedback specialist, who places electrodes on appropriate muscle groups and temperature sensors on a finger, and you are then able to read a dial (or hear a tone) that indicates just how much tension is present. Then the biofeedback specialist will instruct you in just how to relax, or play a relaxation tape, using one of the approaches we have described, and you watch the dial or listen to discover if you are actually relaxing.

At first, patients usually try too hard to relax and actually tense more. You cannot *try* to relax, of course, you can only *let* yourself relax. Trying only makes things worse. You have to let yourself go, allow yourself to relax again as you once were able to as a child. It often takes several training sessions to begin to get the feel of this relaxation and to observe the equipment reflecting the first small relaxation responses. Once the feeling for this comes, learning is much faster. Most people need about a dozen or so sessions to become good enough to be able to continue on their own.

Most biofeedback training consists of one-hour sessions with the equipment, once or twice weekly, with the biofeedback specialist coaching you. But the essential practice is done at home without the equipment, practicing at least twice daily with instructional tapes. When we have done follow-up studies a year later to see how our patients were doing, we found that those who were continuing to practice twice daily with their biofeedback tapes continued to have improved pain control. Those who had quit practicing reported that their pain was as bad as ever—the initial improvement which they reported at the completion of their biofeedback training had been lost.

Pain can occur anywhere in the body. Lois is one of many who have rectal pain. One year ago, at age 43, she underwent a hemorrhoidectomy, and the surgery went smoothly and without complication. But shortly thereafter, Lois began having a deep, aching pain in the rectum. She would be free of pain when she awoke, but with a bowel movement the pain would recur and

Psychological Techniques for Coping with Pain · 119

persist for hours. It was so severe as to prevent her being able to function for three or four hours each day.

She had multiple examinations, barium enemas, lower GI films and CAT scans—all unrevealing. Then a proctologist (rectal surgeon) noted that the levator muscles were in spasm and that Lois had a typical levator ani syndrome. She had some improvement with massage, but the spasms returned.

Lois received biofeedback for levator muscle relaxation training. A rectal probe with a pressure sensor was used to measure the muscle tension, and Lois could see how she would involuntarily tense the muscles in response to stimulation. She was taught how to relax this area and given exercises to practice as well. In just four one-hour sessions Lois was free of pain and has remained so since.

This particular problem, the levator ani syndrome, is surprisingly more common than is generally recognized. It is often thought the pain must be psychogenic if no physical cause (scar, cancer, etc.) can be found. But levator spasm, once identified, can be treated easily with biofeedback.

This brings up an important point often misunderstood by some patients, no matter how often it is explained to them. Biofeedback (or any other relaxation technique) is not a treatment for pain except when tension is the cause of the pain. Biofeedback and other relaxation methods will not cure pain due to nerve damage, adhesions, arthritis, cancer or any similar conditions. These methods are specific pain treatment only when the pain is due to the opposite of relaxation, as in tension states with muscle contraction, constriction of peripheral blood vessels, irritable bowel, headache and similar symptoms.

However, even when these relaxation methods are not specifically aimed at tension-related pain states, they are very effective in eliminating excessive pain caused by tension that accompanies the pain due to other diseases. As we have already described, relaxation is very helpful as part of the psychological approach to pain management. Biofeedback and other relaxation methods help to reduce—not eliminate—the intensity of the pain. Biofeedback seems to be a much more efficient method of relaxation training for those who appear to have lost the voluntary ability to relax and thus do not benefit from the other methods.

But since biofeedback is not in itself going to eliminate your pain—it is not like taking a pain pill and waiting for it to work—you have to work at it. You cannot simply be passive and sit in the biofeedback lab and expect your pain to go away. It is not a treatment that is done to you. It is training you to practice a relaxation skill in which you work at calming your mind and letting go of the tensions in your body. If you learn how to do this and then practice it regularly and faithfully every day, you will eliminate the part of your pain that is due to tension and will be able to keep it away. In some cases this will be all of the pain, but in most cases it will be just a part of it, although a noticeable part that makes a difference.

Pacing Activities

One major effect of the several kinds of relaxation techniques is that they force you to stop everything else for a short time at least twice a day as you slow your body down and enjoy a sense of calm and better self-control. By thus breaking up your day, you are better able to pace your activities.

Let us assume you have decided what you want to do with your life, having made specific goals for work, recreation and social activities. You have a tough mental attitude and angrily refuse to let your pain get in your way. You have started a physical conditioning program to get yourself in the best shape possible and are also learning a relaxation skill. Now you must also learn to "pace" your activities.

This simply means that you must discover how much time you can spend at a task before your pain increases, then learn to stop *before* that happens, taking a break or switching to something else. You will probably be able to increase your time at a task eventually, when you have reached your physical-conditioning goals, but even then there will probably be a point at which further working in the garden or sitting or standing at a workbench will increase your pain. Learning this principle of pacing yourself can be a very useful and practical technique for getting the most out of the day.

Ethel, the "gardening nut," found that if she worked for more than five hours in her garden, she would be bedridden for two or three days.

"At first I would push myself, try to do just a little more. But I would be so sore after that, that I couldn't work at all for several days. This way I watch the time and quit while I'm ahead, and I can work every day. It actually means more hours every week."

Many patients who have pain are in the habit of sitting or lying down a lot because being active causes an increase in pain. But then they become disgusted with themselves and decide to "do something," such as clean the house or work in the yard, and even though they hurt a great deal, they grit their teeth and refuse to quit until they finish the job. Then they are in such severe pain that they must take a lot of analgesics and stay in bed for several days until they recover. They repeat the process of lying around for a while, then plunging into a fierce flurry of work to prove to themselves that they are not cowards or quitters. This may go on for weeks or months. If we were to make a graph of the number of hours they are active each week, it might look like this:

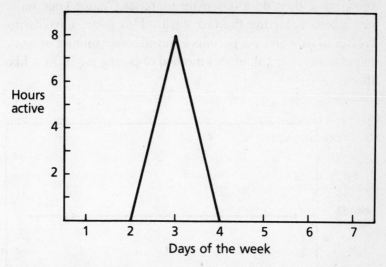

Fig. 2: Poor pacing. The patient gets tired of doing nothing, so forces himself to do a full day's work. The resulting increase of activity puts him down for a week; then the cycle is repeated. This results in only eight hours' work per week.

In this graph, the patient does nothing for several days, recovering from a previous episode of increased pain. Then, in disgust and anger, plunges into some task for a full eight hours in one day, proving to him- or herself that the pain cannot get him or her down. But for the next several days the pain is so much worse that nothing else gets done.

If the pacing principle were followed, patients would experiment to discover how much activity they could perform until the pain *started* to increase. Suppose, for example, that after one hour there was a noticeable increase in pain. That is a signal to stop, and from then on you would watch the clock, or listen for a timer, and stop after forty-five minutes—*before* the pain increased. You would drop everything and lie down for fifteen minutes to practice relaxation ("change your thoughts"), then do a few extra exercises ("move your muscles") before starting the task again. This pattern avoids increases in pain and yet permits a considerable amount of work to get done. A graph of this method of pacing might look like this:

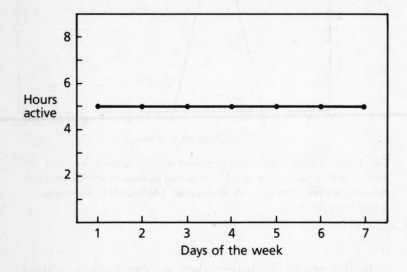

Fig. 3: Proper pacing. The patient has slowly increased his tolerance for work to a maximum of five hours per day. Pain increases if he works longer, so he quits before that happens. This results in thirty-five hours' work per week.

In this graph, the patient may "only" be active for five hours on any one day, because of the frequent breaks, but that amounts to thirty-five hours a week, more than four times better than the "hero" who kills himself for eight hours in a single day and is then bedridden for six days a week.

The important point is to watch the clock or listen for the timer and obey it religiously. This is what permits you to stop and vary your activity in time to avoid a severe flare-up of pain. The kind of break you take is also very important, even if it is only for fifteen minutes. You must definitely change your position completely ("move your muscles") and occupy your mind with something else, such as listening to a relaxation tape and following its instructions ("change your thoughts"). These changes are very restful and restorative.

Most patients discover that as they practice this principle of pacing, they can gradually improve their endurance. For example, after a week or two of working for forty-five minutes and taking a fifteen-minute break, they can then work for fifty minutes and rest for fifteen minutes and still avoid an increase in pain. Then after a week or two of this pattern, they can increase to fifty-five minutes for a week or two, then to one hour, etc. Because they do this very gradually and over a long period of time, they never allow their pain to increase above their tolerance. In pain rehabilitation programs the increase in endurance may occur at a different rate, as you learn to improve your sitting or standing time by just one minute every two or three days. Eventually, of course, a limit will be reached, such as two or three or four hours, after which it will be necessary to stop for a break.

The successful patients work out a schedule and stick to it. Jim, the "bird man" who finally decided not to fool himself, says,

"I have found my limitations and my capability, and I never vary from this program. I take care of my birds, and I've decided that I'm not able to use my body as I used to, so I have taken up college to broaden my knowledge of birds and the science of plants, with the idea of starting a plant hospital. I have regulated my school studies to where it doesn't tear my body down."

* * *

Some skeptical patients say, "Yeah, but who's going to hire you if you have to lie down for fifteen minutes every hour or two?" That's not the point. Would anyone hire you if you lay in bed six days a week? Anyway, is being hired by someone the only reason to get better? This principle permits you to accomplish a great deal more toward *your* goals than you could otherwise, whether you are in business for yourself, working at a hobby, doing chores around the house or visiting with friends. (Yes, you can take breaks when socializing, by changing your position, moving around, etc.)

The patient who insists on being able to work full time, just as before the pain began, or else chooses to do nothing, is usually using the pain as an alibi to get out of doing things he or she can do but doesn't want to do. Pacing your activities permits you to accomplish quite a bit, if you have the motivation and aren't playing games with yourself or others.

Mental Activity

When you "change your thoughts," it need not always be a matter of listening to relaxation tapes or doing some relaxation technique on your own. You can and should do these twice a day, but if you take frequent breaks you will want to have some other mental activity as well so that you can alternate activities and not get bored or stale by repeating the same thing all the time.

You can first of all deliberately direct your train of thought to a different topic altogether when you take your break. Some patients repeat the words of a prayer, or sing a hymn, or plan a trip or project of some kind. From the point of view of controlling your pain, it really doesn't matter what it is you think about, but it obviously should be something that is both interesting and important enough to you that you are willing and able to give it your full attention. The point of engaging in this kind of alternate mental activity is that it is sufficiently absorbing that it completely occupies your attention and takes your mind away from the other task or project you were involved in and are now taking a break from.

The reason for this kind of switching of your attention is that it is necessary to give both your mind and your body a complete rest. It has been found that even when a person is only thinking about an activity, he or she automatically tenses the muscles used in that activity. Therefore, it would not be restful for you to stop and lie down, yet continue to think about the activity while "resting." Just thinking about it would cause you to tighten and tense slightly the very muscles you have been using, and so they would not relax as completely as they could and should. It is necessary for you to think about something completely different in order for your muscles to rest, as well as to provide you with a good mental "change of pace."

Some of us are not very good at directing our thoughts to a different subject. We need to have something outside of us to capture our attention. If that is the case with you, it is perfectly all right to read a book or a magazine on your break, or watch something on television. Or you may listen to some music while you relax or while you do an extra set of your exercises.

Some very enterprising individuals have two or three projects going at the same time. They may do some yard work or household chores, then take a break by doing some work on a hobby, such as painting or ceramics or tying dry flies or woodworking. Then they may sit with their feet up and do some handwork while watching a TV show, then back to the chores or yard work again, and so on. Each change makes a very effective rest and break from the preceding activity. Therefore, the pacing principle is being observed, and a good deal is accomplished without causing an increase in pain.

Emergency Actions

Part of the "move your muscles" approach to pain control involves meeting the need to change what you are doing in order to give tired muscles a break and to produce a new kind of physical stimulation to help block out some of the pain signal. Practicing relaxation techniques, doing physical-conditioning exercises and changing tasks are all effective ways of pacing activities, but, to prevent your pain from getting worse, you must make these changes *before* you get an increase in pain. This is because, as pain gets more severe, it often becomes very difficult to manage. It seems to escape control and get a head start on our attempts to keep it in bounds.

When we allow pain to get out of control like this—or if it does so on its own—all we can do is wait it out and give it time to settle down again. At this time, we need to remember the right mental attitudes we described earlier in the book. It is important not to panic, to remember that these flare-ups have come and gone before, and this flare-up will pass too. And we should have a preplanned routine of things we do to help us through this period—a set of actions we do automatically that help to manage the difficult time when pain is worse than usual.

Marcia, who was hurt in that plane crash, says,
"People provide a distraction from the pain. The minute I'm not busy, I begin to rest more and let down my guard, and the pain starts to get the upper hand. I talk a lot, and that helps me stay on top of the pain."

It is usually *not* helpful to go off by yourself and lie quietly, like a wounded bear. That may be your natural instinct, but it does not provide the physical and mental stimulation which can distract you from your pain. It is better to start an organized sequence of actions that provide a frequent change of pace physically and mentally. Perhaps you may start by lying down with an ice pack or heating pad on the painful area while you listen to one of the relaxation tapes. Next, you go through a set of your conditioning exercises. Then get on the phone and talk to someone about anything but your pain. You may even have an arrangement with a friend that whenever your pain gets out of hand, you can call for an intense and distracting conversation for twenty to thirty minutes or so. Then you may read the Bible or some inspirational literature you have been accumulating for this purpose, after which you may do some exercises again, or listen to another tape or start a writing project, etc.

Work out your own set of things like these to do, and if necessary write them out and put the list up someplace where you can see it. Each time you get a flare-up of pain, check your list and follow it until the episode passes. Having a set pattern of things to do helps greatly, and as you go through the sequence of activities, you may make a brief note about which things seem to help least. You can drop those that do not seem very effective and add actions which are similar to those that are more helpful. Eventually you'll have a very useful list of things to do.

You should know that when you go through a bad time of pain flare-up, there are others who know what you are going through. You are not alone. While you are suffering your pain, around the country and around the world there are other individuals who are also going through a very bad time with quite similar pain. You also need to remember that the episode will pass, the pain will settle down again and you will be able to resume your normal routine. You just need to see it through, to wait it out. This heightened pain will pass as it has before and as it will again in the future. You need to keep busy and distracted so that the time seems to go more quickly. But this flare-up will pass; the pain will blow through you as the wind blows through the trees and then moves on.

So make your list and be prepared so that you will be able to handle these emergencies more effectively. Practice your physical and mental routines each day so that you have these skills readily at hand when you need them (and, of course, practicing them daily makes it more likely that you can avoid flare-ups of pain). Remember that there are plenty of us out there who know what you are going through and are sorry you have to go through it. Remember too that there are new developments in pain research on the horizon, and someday there will be more effective control of chronic pain, perhaps even in our lifetimes. There is reason to be hopeful.

7.
Is It All
in My Head?

Sooner or later almost every person with chronic pain begins to wonder whether he or she is "imagining" the pain, or causing it to happen by some psychological means. This kind of wondering comes about because the pain has continued for a long time, and there has been either no diagnosis made or no response of the pain to treatment. So you begin to wonder, "Am I making this up? Is the pain real or am I imagining it?"

Almost always the pain has a real physical basis. Even in the case of stress reactions causing pain, there is usually muscle tension (sustained tightness of muscle), which accounts for such common pain states as tension headache or backache. Stress reactions can even cause physical activity in the stomach and bowels that result in pain, and these too are "physical" pains rather than "imaginary" pains.

But occasionally, in perhaps 5 percent of the cases of chronic pain (this is my estimate), the pain has a psychological rather than a physical basis. This is a difficult diagnosis to make, and it is also very hard for people to understand why anyone would "want" to feel pain, as if it were being chosen deliberately. In this chapter we will consider the problems of evaluating and understanding *psychogenic pain*—pain resulting from psychological causes.

Making the Diagnosis

Those who have psychogenic pain feel it physically. Wherever it is felt—in the head or chest or back or abdomen—the patient describes it in physical terms. The pain does not have a dreamlike or unreal quality but feels real and physical, and in this regard its description is very similar to the descriptions given by those whose pain is caused by actual or impending tissue injury.

When a person suffering from psychogenic pain seeks medical treatment, the evaluation process is often a lengthy one. The physician will order laboratory studies consistent with his or her evaluation of the most likely cause of the pain symptom as described by the patient, and results of the physical examination. If these studies fail to reveal an adequate explanation for the pain, additional tests may be ordered or specialists asked to consult. These consultants may then request further studies and tests, etc. Only when test after test, and one examination after another, fails to find any significant abnormality to account for the pain is the physician likely to suspect that there might be a psychological basis for it. At this point a psychologist or psychiatrist may be asked to evaluate the patient, or perhaps a pain clinic might be asked to do so.

Psychological evaluation will usually consist of an interview to learn about the patient's background and past history, about present work and family and social circumstances, and whether the patient shows any signs of anxiety or depression or tension, etc. Some psychological tests may be given as well. The psychologist (or psychiatrist) is in the position of evaluating whether the pain *could* be the result of psychological events.

It is important to remember that *not* finding any adequate cause for the pain in the medical evaluation does not by itself prove that the pain is psychogenic, nor does a psychological evaluation that concludes that there are conditions present that *could* account for the pain. The medical evaluation possibly could have missed something. And the findings of the psychological evaluation cannot by themselves rule out a medical basis for the pain. But if both of these conditions are met, namely, that exhaustive medical evaluation is unrevealing and psychological evaluation shows psychological factors possibly or probably accounting for the pain, then the diagnosis of psychogenic pain is very reasonable, and the kind of treatment necessary is clearly psychological.

The logic here is one of ruling out medical causes *and* establishing adequate psychological causes of the pain. Neither approach by itself can make the case, but together they make a case that is very strong. Patients with psychogenic pain sometimes argue with this, thinking that if they feel the pain as physical, then the cause must be physical, and it is the doctor's job to find the physical cause and treat it physically. But in fact, the physician's role is to find the pathology, as it is the patient's "role" to provide the pathology to be found. If that pathology happens to be psychological, then psychological treatment is the answer. And if the patient is really interested in obtaining relief, he or she will be pleased to discover that a cause has been found and will pursue the treatment offered.

Malingering. Aside from the physical disease which is sought, there are other diagnoses to be considered as well. Is the patient malingering? This is always a possibility, although no one likes to admit it. When there are no physical findings to account for the complaint of pain and the complaint is all the physician has to work with, then one of the possible explanations is that the patient is faking. This is rare but not unknown. In order to raise the suspicion of malingering, there must be both the absence of any medical basis for the pain and evidence of an obvious benefit arising from having the pain, a "payoff" that the patient is aware of.

We all remember instances of children having "headaches" or "stomachaches" when they did not want to go to school and high-school girls having "cramps" in order to get out of gym class. Among adults, there are cases of "whiplash" following auto accidents and "back pain" from on-the-job injuries. I have known drug addicts who had "back pain" whenever they could not afford their drugs on the street, and husbands and wives who had various pains whenever they wanted to manipulate the partner's emotions or behavior in some way.

It is always difficult to be sure at first whether malingering is involved. Of course there are genuine cases of whiplash, back pain, cramps, etc., but the physical bases of these are usually obvious. But when there are no signs of physical injury, no muscle spasms, for example, then the question is whether the pain is psychogenic (caused by unconscious psychological mechanisms) or due to malingering (deliberate faking). Once again a psychological or psychiatric evaluation is necessary to determine if it is probable that there are psychological mechanisms involved or if there are more obvious immediate payoffs that the patient is aware of.

Stress Reactions.   As we indicated at the beginning of the chapter, stress reactions are a very common basis for pain complaints. When individuals are under severe and prolonged stress or pressure, many will develop physical symptoms, some of which are painful. Headaches, bowel problems, ulcers, etc., are commonly recognized as being frequently stress related, as are hives, eczema, hypertension, etc. These disorders are now called somatoform, or somatization, disorders. A few years ago they were called psychophysiological stress reactions. And before that they were called psychosomatic illnesses. They all refer to the same process, that of converting stress inputs into physiological dysfunction, *real* physical changes in the body. (Despite common belief, psychosomatic never did mean imaginary.)

These stress reactions are *not* psychogenic, because the bases of the symptoms are genuine physical changes in the body. When pain is part of the complaint, the cause of the pain is usually obvious. In the commonest case of such stress reactions, tension headaches, sustained muscle contractions of the scalp and neck can usually be demonstrated. Similarly, with "irritable," or "functional," bowel dysfunction, the actual motility of the bowel is altered, frequently causing abdominal pain.

In the case of pain related to such somatization, or stress reactions, the physician may also request psychological consultation. This is not so much to identify psychological causes or help with diagnosis (as in the case of psychogenic pain), because the diagnosis is often obvious; rather it is to help identify the sources of stress and to help teach the patient better ways of handling the stress. There is a psychological specialty called behavioral medicine which has developed very efficient techniques for stress management. These techniques are quite similar to those we describe for pain control.

These, then, are the major possibilities for diagnosis if there is no medical disease found to underlie the symptom of pain: the pain can be due to a stress reaction—somatization; it can be a false complaint—malingering; or it can be due to unconscious mental mechanisms—psychogenic. It is this last that we will examine a little more closely as it is less well understood than the others.

How Psychogenic Pain Can Occur

There are two serious mental disorders in which pain can arise as a symptom, but these are far less prevalent than other causes of psychogenic pain. A psychotic patient can *hallucinate* the pain—for example, believing that extraterrestrials are sending torture rays into his or her body, the patient feels the pain of this. This hallucination (false perception) is equivalent to hearing voices or seeing things that are not there. It is not common, but it can occur.

Another patient, seriously depressed, may have a *delusion* about his or her body, believing it is rotting, for example, and feels pain as a part of this. About 50 percent of all hospitalized depressed patients complain of pain, although often it is a minor complaint, and the pain is usually part of some delusion (false belief) relating to the body.

But the existence of psychogenic pain does not necessarily mean that the person is hallucinating or delusional and suffering severe mental illness. In fact, the chances are that it is a much less serious kind of somatoform disorder called a conversion reaction. This is an interesting process in which either sensations or movements are dramatically altered as a way of compensating for some intense emotion. There are certain personality types that are more likely than others to use this process unconsciously, but almost anyone can have it happen at one time or another.

Examples of conversion reactions I have seen lately are: a sudden loss of voice; a loss of feeling (numbness) on one side of the body *(not* due to a stroke); a sudden and temporary deafness and a dramatic uncoordination of the legs, making walking almost impossible. Others have reported cases of blindness and paralysis as well. Usually these afflictions are referred to as "hysterical blindness," "hysterical deafness," etc., because the personality type most likely to develop these symptoms was formerly called hysteric (now called histrionic). But it is probably better to speak of "conversion blindness" or "psychogenic deafness," etc., because other personality types also develop these symptoms on occasion.

Martha is 64 and complains of burning on one side of her face. It feels like a stinging, burning pain. She has had it for forty-one years. Doctors had never been able to find an explanation. No analgesic had ever had any effect nor had any other medication.

What happened when Martha was 23 years old? She found out that her husband was having an affair. "It was like a slap in the face," she says.

Martha had a difficult time in therapy. It was nearly impossible to have her relive the emotion she experienced on learning of her husband's infidelity forty-one years earlier. Even under hypnosis, she could only recount the event without feeling, as though she were a mere observer. The stinging, burning pain in her cheek did not lessen, but she did seem to become less concerned about it. She stopped mentioning the pain and did not seem to think about it unless asked about it. When she left the clinic, Martha was in a good mood.

"I guess I'll always have this pain," she said, "but it doesn't bother me anymore. Even if it's in my imagination, I guess I can live with it."

Martha needed to keep her pain as a way of remembering always how she had been wronged. But she was comfortable with this now and no longer felt a need to pursue a medical solution to her pain.

These symptoms usually develop as a response to a particularly difficult situation that arouses an intense emotion which is more than the person can bear—and there is no way out. The symptom occurs suddenly, and almost magically it resolves the entire situation for the patient.

For example, a woman who experienced sudden and temporary deafness had this occur at a train station as she arrived home from vacation. A relative told her that a manic-depressive sister of the patient's had just moved into town and would need looking after, as the patient had done for years in the past. The poor woman could not bear to hear this news and suddenly lost her hearing. She had to leave home again to go to a distant clinic to get help for her "deafness"—and so escaped the difficult situation at least temporarily. Although this process seems obvious to us in reviewing the story, it was not at all apparent to the patient at the time. That is what is so interesting about these symptoms—the mind apparently produces them quite automatically and unconsciously, without the patient's awareness.

On a number of occasions I have seen men who had a "weakness" or "partial paralysis" of an arm, with accompanying pain in the hand and arm. In each case it began in a situation in which the man wanted to punch a supervisor or boss, so enraged was he over an incident that had occurred. The pain and paralysis prevented the violence, which he did not dare allow, and it also got him out of the situation.

In most such cases there are several common elements which we can piece together. There is first a very difficult and stressful situation from which there is no easy way out. The woman who became deaf could not move away from the sister who plagued her. The worker could not afford to punch his boss. And yet in each case the impulse was so strong as to be nearly irresistible.

Second, the emotion aroused by the situation is usually very intense, whether it is panic or rage or sexual lust or wanting to give up responsibilities and be taken care of—whatever. These emotions are not only very strong but also very uncomfortable to have because they are not really "acceptable": the person does not want to feel them or recognize that he or she has strong feelings of this sort. We usually like to think of ourselves as "nice" people, and nice people are not overcome by such feelings as these.

Third, and usually quite suddenly, the problem is solved by the appearance of the symptom. The individual goes blind or deaf or becomes paralyzed or has pain. The intense uncomfortable feeling disappears, the person is taken out of the situation and the symptom itself seems to symbolize the entire conflict situation the patient was in. The paralyzed arm cannot punch, the deaf ears cannot hear the bad news, the lost voice cannot say the terrible things the person wanted to say, etc. In hindsight, in the simplified telling of the story, it all seems very obvious, but it usually takes quite a bit of detective work to put all the pieces together.

One of the interesting features of these psychogenic symptoms, including psychogenic pain, is that the patient who comes in with the symptoms usually seems to be fairly calm about it. You might think that if you suddenly went blind or deaf or paralyzed or had severe pain, you would be very upset and distressed and fairly desperate to have something done about it. But these patients do not seem distressed at all. Although they are asking for relief, they seem calm, almost bland about the whole thing. They give the impression of being in a comfortable emotional balance with the symptom, as though it really is solving something for them. This is called "la belle indifference."

No wonder the usual pain treatments don't work for these patients—such treatments are simply irrelevant. The patients cannot afford to get better until an acceptable alternative, a better way out than the symptom, is available. And once the better way out is found, they are usually quite well. Occasionally, some face-saving other treatment is helpful, but if psychological treatment does not occur, other methods are usually of no use.

Another cause of psychogenic pain needs to be mentioned,

although it is even less common than the conversion reaction. This is *hypochondriasis*. Hypochondriasis refers to a fascinated absorption in the experience of illness, a condition of being so involved in one's own sickness that there is almost an inability to think of, or be emotionally involved in, very much else.

There are basically three kinds of hypochondriasis, although any patient might have one or two or all three kinds. The simplest is that of being focused on many physical symptoms. This means noticing many bodily sensations and worrying about them, wondering what they mean and suspecting that there may be some disease causing the sensations.

The second type of hypochondriasis is called disease phobia, which refers to the fear of getting a serious illness. This is not common, but there are those who will not touch doorknobs or shake hands with others, nor use public toilet facilities, etc., for fear of becoming infected with some dreaded disease—cancer or AIDS or whatever. Such persons are usually exceptionally clean and neat, much more conscious of health habits and diet than others are, and in general they spend a lot of time and energy trying to avoid one or more specific diseases of which they are frightened.

The third kind of hypochondriasis is the type in which the person is convinced that he or she has some very serious disease despite medical evaluation and reassurance to the contrary. This is probably the rarest kind of all, except when part of one of the more serious mental illnesses, because such a belief in the face of contrary evidence borders on being delusional.

Most pain patients whose pain is of physical origin become, over a period of time, somewhat hypochondriacal. This is because the pain makes them so conscious of their bodies that they start noticing and worrying about other physical symptoms too. And when the pain persists, they start suspecting they may have some serious disease which no one has found yet—or why would the pain be there?

On the other hand, a true hypochondriac, though he or she does not have a physical cause for pain, may worry so about symptoms that they are magnified and may become painful. Or he or she may be so certain that a terrible disease is present, or so frightened of one, that ordinary sensations are similarly magnified and become painful. Sometimes this kind of hypochondriasis with psychogenic pain is associated with depression, but other times it is not and appears as a separate psychological disorder in its own right. When it comes with depression, then treating the depression usually also solves the hypochondriasis and psychogenic pain too. When the hypochondriasis and accompanying psychogenic pain are the chief problem, then psychotherapy is necessary, sometimes aided by certain psychiatric medications.

Treatment of Psychogenic Pain

As we mentioned earlier, patients with psychogenic pain are often reluctant to see a psychologist because they feel the pain is physical and want a medical diagnosis and treatment. But if evaluation shows no medical pathology, and evidence of psychological "pathology" is present, then the treatment needs to be psychological.

The psychological treatment for conversion pain is psychotherapy. It consists of exploring the life situation in which the pain symptom arose. What was going on when the symptom began? What was the situation at work? At home? What were the emotions the patient was feeling at the time? In psychotherapy, the situation is safe: the patient can safely relive the intense situation and unbearable emotions. The relationship between the symptom and the emotions and conflict situation becomes apparent, the unconscious mechanisms become conscious and the patient is then able to work out what happened and find a more acceptable, useful alternative.

All of this is said and summarized very quickly here, but obviously it takes time. Sometimes the therapy can be done in just one or a few sessions, and sometimes it may take a number of weeks or months. It all depends on how difficult the life situation of the patient is, whether the symptom arose from a single incident or developed over time as a culmination of a very complicated family or work relationship problem. But the conversion symptom, the pain itself, often disappears quickly as the therapy gets under way, and may not even be noticed by the patient as attention is focused on the more serious issues that gave rise to it.

In the case of hypochondriasis, the success of treatment is much less certain because the patients are usually much more resistant to psychological therapy. They are either so worried about medical matters or so convinced that the problem is a medical one, that they resist any attempts at explanation and reassurance.

The treatment of hypochondriasis is also difficult because the causes of the disorder are quite variable from case to case. And almost always it develops slowly over many months or years, not suddenly. There is no simple formula such as: intense emotion + difficult situation = symptom that allows escape, as there is in the case of conversion symptoms. There is one element which is commonly present, and that is a kind of emotional isolation in which the patient has weakened ties with others and so seems to fuss over his or her own health the way a mother fusses over her child. This seems a kind of substitute for a normal caring relationship. But this is frequently only a clue and not necessarily the whole story, so psychotherapy (if the patient agrees to it at all) is sometimes long and tedious as things get pieced together.

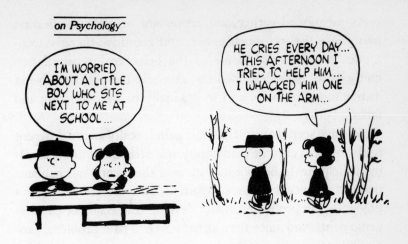

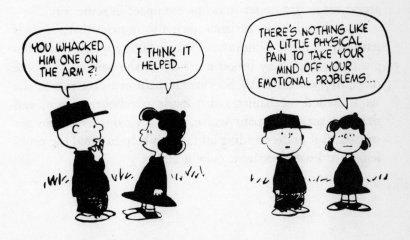

Fig. 4: Somatization. Some persons have pain for psychological reasons—
"psychogenic pain." Even more commonly, those with physically caused
pains may focus on them to avoid having to deal with emotional stresses or
problems with others.

Is It All in My Head? · 143

As mentioned earlier, antidepressant or other medication may make the job much easier, and cognitive-therapy techniques together with some of the behavioral rehabilitation methods we have described can also help the patient to begin to live more normally and so gradually to start thinking and feeling better.

We have seen that psychogenic pain is really a very different problem from chronic pain of physical origin, but understanding it helps us to be aware of some of the mental mechanisms that can also occur in chronic-pain patients. People who have a physical-pain problem can also develop conversion or psychogenic pain. And since they already have a pain problem, producing a new symptom is not necessary—just a sudden worsening of the pain which already exists can get them out of a difficult situation. Many chronic-pain patients themselves have noticed that their pain gets much worse if they have an argument or are under stress or are upset in some way.

And chronic-pain patients have also noticed that, as their pain makes them withdraw and their family relationships begin to weaken, they brood more about the pain and become more hypochondriacal. So chronic pain can give rise to the same mental mechanisms that cause psychogenic pain, and that can make the pain worse, and a vicious cycle can get started. But understanding all this can help to avoid the problem or at least alleviate it once it starts.

8.
About Analgesics—
and Alternatives

The strong prescription analgesics, which are such a blessing for those with acute pain following injury or surgery, or in certain diseases, are a source of trouble and even danger for those with chronic pain. When used over a long time, tolerance and dependence and addiction develop (these are not the same). These drugs cloud the mind, cause constipation and other gastrointestinal symptoms, make depression worse and are habit-forming. Their long-term effects on liver and kidneys have not become clear, but there is more than suspicion that they cause problems here as well, especially when combined with nonprescription analgesics.

Tolerance to narcotics occurs in large measure as a biochemical event. The more you take and the longer you take them, the more your liver develops the enzymes to neutralize the effects of the narcotics. With repeated use, there is also a change that occurs within cells. The net effect is that the drugs become less and less effective over time. Many patients have found that, whereas one codeine tablet (let's say) would almost eliminate the pain initially, now three or four are not as effective as one was—although the side effects may be greater. This is tolerance, and it is a worrisome problem to most pain patients and their doctors.

Part of the problem arises from the fact that these strong analgesics were given initially when the pain was acute (still new) and simply continued as the pain persisted. And as those who have pain naturally want to escape their suffering, they want the analgesics that provide the most relief. But although that is quite appropriate for the acute-pain state, it is a mistake to continue this approach when the pain becomes chronic. It is safer to find the *weakest* analgesics, which just barely take the edge off the pain, in order to avoid developing tolerance and other complications.

Dependence on analgesics refers to the fact that when narcotics have been used a great deal, if they are suddenly discontinued, withdrawal symptoms appear. Under usual circumstances these consist of tremors, diarrhea and cramps, runny nose and feelings of jitteriness. But most pain patients do not experience these symptoms to a great extent if they stop taking their analgesics for a few days. And since they hardly ever have a "craving" for the drug either (which is what is meant by *addiction*), it is hard for most patients to believe that they are dependent on their pain pills. What they do notice is that their pain gets much worse when they leave off taking the pills, and this seems to them to be proof that they only take their pills because of pain and not addiction, that they need their analgesics but are not dependent on them.

Although this seems logical, and it is understandable that those with chronic pain believe this—and worry a good deal that the doctors will misunderstand and cut off their only means of pain control—in fact it doesn't work this way. The test of quitting the drugs for a few days isn't adequate, but even if it were, the question is not whether dependence or addiction has developed but rather what is the most effective means of controlling the pain. (In fact there *are* ways of taking narcotics for pain control without dependence or addiction developing—and without tolerance occurring as well, although this is more difficult to avoid. But these are not the only problems.)

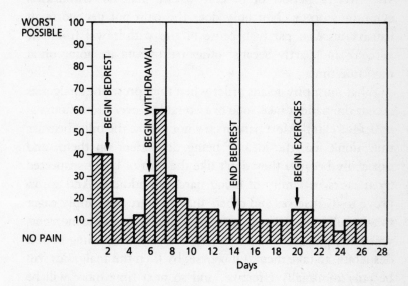

Fig. 5: Withdrawal. This patient experienced a marked worsening of his pain following an abrupt quitting of his narcotics. This was the chief withdrawal symptom. Within a few days his pain level fell dramatically. It was even possible to begin exercising without worsening of the pain. His pain had been his body's signal of the need for the analgesic.

In the graph shown here, we have an example of how pain can be maintained at an abnormally high level because of the problem of narcotic dependence. When this patient quit his analgesics abruptly ("cold turkey"), his chief symptom of withdrawal was a marked worsening of his pain. After the withdrawal period, his residual pain was much less than it had been previously when he was still taking the narcotics. This is not an isolated case—we have seen this happen to others as well. Almost all pain treatment centers, however, wean patients off their analgesics slowly, tapering the dose so gradually over a period of several weeks that no withdrawal symptoms occur. Not only does the pain not get worse, it usually lessens, partly because of the withdrawal from the narcotic and partly because other treatments are going on at the same time.

What most physicians order when they prescribe analgesics is that the patient take "one or two tablets every four hours *as needed* for pain." Most patients try not to take the pills, because they don't like the idea of being dependent on them, and especially because they don't like the idea of being suspected by doctors or family of being narcotics addicts. And so, to prove to themselves and others that they are not simply eager to take pills, the patients wait until the last possible moment, when the pain is very severe and they are beginning to feel desperate, to take them. Of course, by then the analgesics will be only minimally effective, and so next time more will be needed to provide pain relief. Ultimately, this pattern combined with the tolerance effect will cause larger and larger doses to be required.

Melanie is 28 years old and works as a securities clerk at a local bank. She has constant severe headaches, beginning with a tightness in the neck and spreading over her head. At times the pain is a throbbing in the temples so severe her vision blurs and she has difficulty thinking.

Melanie knows the headaches are related to job stress because they began only after she had been on this fast-paced, hectic job involving millions of dollars for a few months. Like many others who work under such pressure, Melanie began smoking and drinking a lot of coffee. However, she likes her job because it is a real challenge and is always different.

She began taking a lot of aspirin to control these headaches, but that didn't help much and was upsetting her stomach. Her doctor then prescribed a muscle relaxant, and a moderate-strength narcotic, Percocet. Melanie found that the muscle relaxant made her very sleepy, so she stopped taking it, but the Percocet made her headaches quite tolerable. However, over a period of several months she had found it necessary to increase the amount from one tablet four times a day to two, and sometimes three tablets, four times daily. Her doctor became alarmed and insisted that she visit a pain clinic as he would no longer prescribe the medication.

After evaluation to be sure that her headaches were indeed tension headaches and nothing more serious, Melanie has started a rehabilitation program. She began biofeedback training for relaxation of the neck and scalp muscles, a physical-therapy program for muscle stretching and strengthening, and aerobic conditioning to help discharge stress and tension. At the same time she has discontinued drinking coffee and is attending an evening support group for help in quitting smoking. She has been given a withdrawal schedule to follow to taper off the Percocet and is already feeling much better.

"I'm almost completely off the pills, and I'm amazed at how much brighter I feel," Melanie said. "I didn't realize that I was in such a fog. I've only just started the biofeedback and physical therapy, but my headaches are already not as severe as they were. It's absolutely incredible, but I'm taking less pain medication and the headaches are going away."

The Conditioned Pain Response

Most doctors as well as patients are not aware of how taking analgesics on an "as-needed" basis can cause the pain itself to increase by becoming conditioned to the body's need for the analgesics. This usually does not become manifest in treating the short-term acute pains but develops over a period of months.

Here is how it happens—how it could happen to you. You wait until the pain is severe and take the pill. This causes a lessening of the pain, and anything which lessens the pain is a positive reinforcer, that is, becomes sought after. So the next time the pain is severe—whether in a few hours or days—you are more likely to take the pill again. And the pattern is repeated, again and again: increase in pain—take the pain pill; increase in pain—take the pill, etc.

Gradually, tolerance and dependence develop, as we have described. One pill no longer does the job, so two are needed to reduce the pain—a sign of increasing tolerance. And as the dosages are increased, a corresponding dependence develops—the tendency for withdrawal symptoms to appear when the analgesic is stopped. But as we have already noted, and the graph on page 147 shows, the withdrawal symptom most likely to appear is an increase in pain. The pain becomes more severe as a signal to replenish the supply of narcotics which the body has now come to need.

This is how it looks in outline form:

1. Increase in pain—take analgesic tablet

2. Increase in pain—take analgesic tablet, etc.

3. Tolerance develops, so

4. Increase in pain—take two analgesic tablets, etc.

5. Dependence develops, so

6. Physical need for analgesics (withdrawal)—increase in pain.

This is not an uncommon pattern. It happens to most pain patients who use narcotics every day for pain control. Unfortunately, it is usually difficult to explain the problem to them in a way they can understand and accept. To the patients, it seems that they take the pills because they hurt, and it is hard for them to believe that they hurt more because they take the pills. When some patients hear this explanation, they think they are being told that the pain is all in their head. Others think that they are being accused of being addicts. Both of these ideas are incorrect, of course—their problem is physical pain worsened by physical withdrawal; there is no addiction in the sense of "craving" the drug.

But there is now ample clinical evidence from many pain centers that simply taking the analgesics on a regular by-the-clock basis, such as every four hours, can prevent the increase in pain due to the withdrawal signal. And then the gradual tapering of the dosage actually leads to a reduction in pain. It is hard for patients to understand why they hurt more when they took more analgesics and hurt less after they withdrew from them, but this is very common and they don't quarrel with the results.

Now that we have considered the problems that come with relying on narcotic analgesics for pain control, let's consider the practical and effective ways of managing pain with analgesics.

How to Use Analgesics

When it is clear that your pain is not going to go away, you should start treating it like chronic pain. You will have to discuss these principles with your prescribing physician, of course, and work out a plan that is appropriate in your case.

First of all, as we mentioned earlier, you need to take the weakest analgesic which just "takes the edge off" the pain. In acute pain, the goal is to be as comfortable as possible for the short duration of the pain—a few days or weeks. But when the pain appears likely to be indefinite, then it is necessary to change to a weaker dose or a weaker analgesic in order to avoid the development of tolerance and its associated complications.

Second, unlike the "as-needed" schedule, which was appropriate for the short-term pain state, it is necessary now to change to a fixed schedule of taking the analgesics in order to avoid the "peaks and valleys" of inconsistent analgesia and to avoid the conditioned pain response as well. Let's describe this more specifically.

Once the weakest effective analgesic is found (it should *not* eliminate the pain, only reduce it slightly), it should be taken regularly, by the clock, whether the pain is severe or not, in order to keep the pain at a more consistent level. If you wait until your pain is severe (because you're afraid of becoming addicted), you will find the pain very difficult to control at all and be on your way to escalating the dose.

The principle here is really like pacing yourself again. You need to stay ahead of the pain and keep it from increasing, using the minimal amount of analgesic necessary to do so. It is much safer and more effective to take a weak analgesic in a fixed amount and to follow the clock religiously. There are now thousands of patients who were once taking the equivalent of eight to ten codeine tablets daily and still hurting a lot, who are actually having less pain and taking only one or two aspirin (or aspirin substitute) three or four times daily—or taking nothing at all for pain.

The problem with the strong analgesics, as we have described, is that as you develop tolerance and the drug becomes less effective, your pain seesaws a great deal. A typical graph for many patients who either wait as long as they can to take their analgesic or who develop tolerance to the narcotic would look like this:

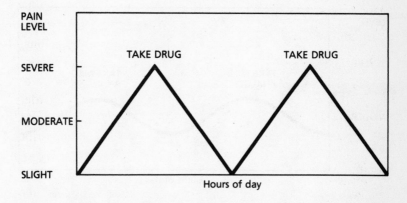

Fig. 6: Inconsistent pain control. This is due to waiting for pain to be very severe before taking the analgesic, then needing a strong narcotic to get relief.

Here you can see the "peaks and valleys" of inconsistent analgesia. There is only slight pain when the analgesic is first taken but severe pain before it is taken again, and so there are frequent wide swings in pain intensity. If you followed this schedule, you might be very comfortable and possibly oversedated when the pain is slight and then very uncomfortable and unable to function when the pain is severe. The constant swing from slight to severe and back again is exhausting and disruptive.

Patients who learn to take weaker analgesics more frequently on a fixed schedule enjoy two advantages: they do not develop a tolerance for strong narcotics, so in case of emergency they can obtain relief of very severe pain; and they avoid the daily increases in pain to severe levels. If you follow this plan, your graph should look like this:

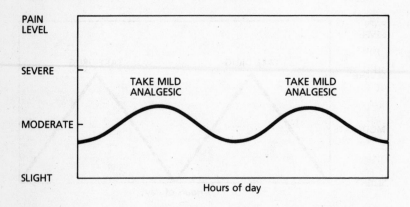

Fig. 7: Consistent pain control. Pain level can be kept moderate by using a mild analgesic and following a strict time schedule.

Here you see that the pain level fluctuates only slightly, staying at the moderate level. At this level you can still function, and because there are not the great swings in pain intensity, you can pace yourself and plan your day appropriately. It is much easier to deal with a constant level of pain than one that is always changing, especially when the pain is not severe.

We suggested earlier that it is better not to take any narcotics at all for chronic pain because of the complications which develop. It is usually better to take one of the nonprescription analgesics, which we will describe below. Most pain patients scoff at the idea of "taking two aspirin," and in fact there are many kinds of pain states that are not at all helped by any amount of nonprescription analgesic. But there are also many that can be helped, if these weaker analgesics are used properly.

"I found the clock schedule really works," Jim says. "It was rough the first week because my pain really shot up; I think it must have been the withdrawal. But then when I got the junk out of my system, my pain level actually fell a little. I used to think I could take aspirin by the handful and it wouldn't touch my pain, but that's because I'd wait too long to take something. Now I take two aspirins every four hours, and it keeps the pain from getting out of hand, if I pace myself right.

"Sometimes I feel foolish taking the aspirin when I'm not hurting worse but it's time to, but I learned that if I don't I'll pay for it later. I wouldn't go near the hard stuff now for anything."

Nonprescription Analgesics
We mentioned in Chapter 4 that there really are just three kinds of nonprescription analgesics: aspirin, acetaminophen (e.g., Tylenol) and ibuprofen (e.g., Nuprin). All of them seem to have the effect of controlling pain by inhibiting the activity in the nerve endings that normally start signaling pain. These analgesics are especially helpful in taking the edge off mild-to-moderate pain, as from tension headache, sore muscles, joint pain, etc. Aspirin and ibuprofen are more effective if inflammation is part of the cause of pain, which is frequently the case in muscle and joint pains. Ibuprofen is less irritating to the stomach and gut than is aspirin.

It is important to follow the directions on the label, or your physician's instructions. Just because these medicines can be bought without prescription does not mean that they should be used carelessly. I have seen a number of patients who had chronic gut problems triggered by ulcers caused by excessive aspirin use. Kidney disease is well reported as a result of overuse of aspirin, and excessive use of acetaminophen has been reported to cause liver disease. Using ibuprofen to excess can also cause gut symptoms. So follow directions, staying within the guidelines of using no more than one or two tablets every four hours. And if that amount does not have any effect on your pain, don't take any.

In the long run, you will probably have to stop taking aspirin or acetaminophen or ibuprofen for the same reason you must discontinue the narcotics—because long-continued use (like large amounts) can be quite harmful, and you may not discover this until it is too late.

In long-term pain, analgesics almost always become a part of the problem rather than an effective treatment. This is because they are really meant only for the control of short-term, acute pain. The great majority of pain patients who have succeeded in overcoming their pain handicap, who have learned to live well with their pain, have given up on pain pills altogether. Contrariwise, those pain patients who use analgesics regularly and do not give them up do least well in pain treatment programs, do not function well at all and tend to develop other problems—both medical and psychological—because of the analgesics.

Quitting Drugs

If you want to stop using nonprescription analgesics, simply do so. There is no significant withdrawal or rebound problem to worry about. No matter how many you may have been taking each day, nor for how long, you can stop abruptly with no ill effects. You may miss the habit of taking pills, but that is probably all you'll notice.

Narcotics are another matter, however. In pain treatment clinics patients are detoxified (withdrawn) slowly, over a matter of some weeks. If you stop abruptly, you are likely to notice a sudden sharp increase in pain and perhaps other withdrawal symptoms, which are also unpleasant. It depends greatly on how large an amount of the opiate drug you were dependent on. But in pain centers your usual dose is likely to be reduced by approximately 10 percent every two days or so, so that you experience none of these withdrawal effects.

It is a lot easier to withdraw from the drugs when you have other tools for controlling the pain, and of course those are the reasons for going to pain clinics or treatment centers. We have been describing these tools or techniques right along—the physical conditioning and psychological techniques of pain control—and there are enough alternatives available to make analgesic withdrawal quite feasible.

If you cannot get to a treatment facility, it would be a good idea to take several steps before you start withdrawing from narcotics. First, discuss your plan with your prescribing physician. Second, begin the training in the physical and psychological techniques for pain control we described in the previous chapters. Third, as you begin to acquire skills in these techniques, begin tapering off the analgesics.

The way to taper off or withdraw is to be sure that you are taking your usual daily amount of pain pills at fixed times, by the clock, without any variation. For example, if you usually take 2 codeine tablets at a time, averaging 8 per day, then take them at regular times, such as 8:00 A.M., noon, 4:00 P.M., and 8:00 P.M. Then, take ½ tablet less every other day, meaning you take 7½ tablets for two days, then 7 tablets for two days, then 6½, etc. You break or cut them in half to get the dose just right.

It doesn't matter at which of the times you choose to reduce the amount first. Pick the time your pain is least troublesome—it may be the morning, when you have been less active, or the evening, when you have had several codeine tablets already during the day—but it really doesn't matter where you start. After two weeks you'll be taking only one tablet four times a day, and in another two weeks you'll have stopped altogether.

I have found that most patients have no difficulty in following such a schedule and experience no withdrawal symptoms. The majority notice no worsening of their pain and feel very much brighter. After they have stopped their analgesics, they realize how mentally sluggish or dull they had been before without having been aware of it. They usually feel better physically, as well.

The TENS Alternative

We discussed the use of TENS (transcutaneous electrical nerve stimulation) previously, in Chapter 4, but it is worth mentioning again here because for many patients it seems to be a relatively safe and effective alternative to analgesics, especially for the long-term management of pain.

TENS seems to work both by blocking injury signals directly in the periphery of the body and also by stimulating descending inhibition of the incoming injury signals in the spine. It works best in cases where the pain is well localized, such as in a foot, or a compression fracture of the spine—in some hospitals it is used routinely for postoperative pain control—but it can also be helpful with pains in larger areas.

The success of TENS is greatly improved if it is part of the entire treatment program described in this book. When used by itself, without undertaking the other pain-control techniques, including withdrawal from analgesics, the rate of success of TENS is moderate at best—about a 50 percent success rate initially, declining to about 30 percent after one year. But when it is used along with all the other methods of pain control, then TENS' success rate increases to about 65 percent initially, declining to about 50 percent after one year.

These success rates are averages of results of a number of old studies that were not well controlled, that used different standards to judge "success" and TENS devices that are primitive by today's standards—so the figures are only rough estimates.

Harvey, age 73, has had his left leg amputated above the knee because of vascular disease. However, he has phantom pain, that is, he feels the same pain in the missing leg as he felt before the amputation. He has had this problem—one which about 10 percent of amputees have—for seventeen years now, and he is quite worn out by it.

Surgeons have operated on Harvey's stump to remove neuromas, with no benefit. He has tried many different analgesics and antidepressants, with no benefit. He has had many nerve blocks, which only made the pain worse.

A TENS device was tried, with electrodes placed on the stump over the main nerve pathways. Harvey could feel the electric tingling going into his phantom leg. Almost immediately, the pain stopped. In the past several weeks, he has found that the pain would stay away for longer periods after he took the TENS off. Now he uses it for a half-hour twice a day and has not had any pain at all for about a month.

"How long have these things been around?" Harvey asks.

"About fifteen years now," I tell him.

Harvey looks very serious and angry. "Do you mean that I've been suffering for all these years when I could have been wearing one of these all along?" he asks. "Why did I have all those nerve blocks and surgeries? Why didn't they try one of these things first?" He thumps his fist on my desk.

I just look at Harvey and shrug. "How're you feeling now?" I ask him.

He hesitates, then relaxes and grins widely. "Like a new man," he said. "The hell with them. That's all in the past. I've got some living to catch up on."

TENS requires a prescription. If you have not tried a TENS device for your pain, discuss this with your physician. And find a knowledgeable professional, such as a physical therapist or registered nurse who is experienced with these devices and can show you how to use one. Not all kinds of pain are responsive to TENS, but it is certainly worth a try. It is quite safe, although it cannot be used by someone whose cardiac pacemaker is not shielded against the TENS frequencies. Some individuals have sensitive skin, which may be irritated by the stimulating electrodes—but this is the only common side effect and can be controlled by discontinuing stimulation or changing electrode position or type of electrode.

A sensible attitude is necessary when using TENS or any other pain-control technique: do not expect magic, but do not have a negative attitude, either. Keep an open mind and observe the effect carefully. If after a few days you are not sure if TENS helps, try using it every other day and compare how you feel with it and without it. A two- to four-week trial is usually enough.

And remember also that TENS is just one more method of several which you need to use together for best results. You need to have goals that you are working toward; you need to exercise regularly so you can do easily the things you want to do; you need to learn one of the mental pain-control techniques and practice it regularly and to pace your activities throughout the day. And, as we have said, you need to withdraw from analgesics to avoid the problems associated with their long-term use, just as you stop caffeine and nicotine to avoid their effects of increasing irritability and tension. No one of these things may produce a dramatic effect by itself, but when you combine them all you should notice a significant improvement in your ability to cope with pain—and that's what this is all about.

9.
How to Manage Cancer Pain

There are some important differences between the ways of managing pain due to cancer (or other terminal disease), and managing the nonfatal pain states we have been referring to so far in this book. But there are also some similarities in the methods of controlling both classes of pain. In this chapter we describe what is special about the pain management techniques as applied to terminal diseases and what a total pain management program might consist of for patients with such diseases. But first we need to consider what is the nature of this pain.

Myths Versus Facts

One of the reasons cancer is a frightening disease is that it is sometimes thought that it is always associated with terrible pain. This fear of suffering terribly is usually more upsetting than the idea of dying. It is not death but pain that worries us. Many people talk about the *quality* of life when they discuss their illness, rather than the length of life. And by this they mean that they can, if they must, come to terms with dying, before their time, but they don't want to suffer.

But cancer and other terminal diseases are not always associated with pain. In one large study conducted in a distinguished U.S. cancer center, only about 38 percent of cancer patients receiving treatment for their disease had pain. Of those whose condition was terminal, about 60 percent had pain requiring attention.

The likelihood of pain with cancer depends upon the kind of cancer and the stage of the disease. Only about 5 percent of those in the early stages of cancer have any pain, and where pain is present, it is in connection with the kinds with solid tumors. As the disease progresses, there is an increase in the chances of having pain, to an average of about 40 percent for most of those receiving treatment. Finally, in the terminal stages, the probability of pain ranges from 60 to 70 percent in several reported studies.

Another common myth is that cancer pain is always terrible, causing a great deal of agonized suffering. In the 1960s a study of hospitalized cancer patients showed that they felt their world to be one of alien and meaningless and unpredictable pain, with no end in sight, and that the pain caused them to withdraw from interest in the world and their families. It was a life with the qualities of a nightmare, showing how poorly treated cancer pain could indeed cause a great deal of agony and suffering.

But in the years since, a great deal has been learned about pain control in cancer (and similarly fatal illnesses), and such uncontrolled pain should no longer occur. In a large study in the Midwest, it appeared that the average person thinks cancer is more painful than the patients themselves report. Inpatients with metastatic cancer reported their pain as no more severe than did outpatients with rheumatoid arthritis, and *less* severe than the pain reported by outpatients in a pain clinic for other pain problems.

Most persons with cancer can now expect to live a relatively long time, on the order of years, between the time of their diagnosis and the time of their death. For some types of cancer this is because of great improvements in treatment; for others it is because of earlier diagnoses than in the past. However, the important point is that, unlike what many persons believe, cancer patients spend most of their remaining time living just as usual, going on about their daily routines much as they have always done, except for the interruptions caused by receiving cancer therapy, and for the emotional distress caused by knowing they have a serious illness. Cancer patients most certainly do not have to take to their beds when they receive the diagnosis, and suffer severe pain for all their remaining days, as some persons may imagine.

Part of the great improvement in pain control in cancer has come from better understanding of the cancer diseases themselves. Treatment of the underlying disease in any case—directing therapy to the area of tumor involvement, for example—can reduce or eliminate the pain associated with the spread, or metastasis, of tumor to healthy tissue. For example, there is often more pain associated with bone cancer or metastasis of tumor to bone than with other kinds of cancer. But radiation given to the involved area can shrink or eliminate the tumor at the site and reduce or eliminate the pain.

Another part of the great improvement in pain control in cancer has to do with the great advances in knowledge about pain mechanisms in general and the advance in pain-control techniques in particular. There have been developments in surgical techniques that are very useful, particularly for terminal patients, and there are a number of kinds of nerve-block and radiation treatments, which, while not advisable for patients whose pain is not associated with malignant disease, are exceptionally helpful in treating those with cancer or other malignant pain.

Finally, another major advance in cancer pain control has come from the hospice movement and spread to other areas of medicine as well. Attention to humanitarian concerns has been shown to be a very important element of care. This means recognition of the person as an individual, respect for his or her dignity and wishes, and giving the person the opportunity to talk about his or her fears and other emotional reactions. But the hospice movement, especially in Great Britain, has also shown how it is possible to provide excellent pain control in cancer with proper use of analgesics. The application of these psychological and analgesic techniques to the care of patients with cancer is now widespread and has largely eliminated the nightmarish existence during the terminal stages which was so common just a generation ago.

Evaluation

There are several causes of cancer pain, just as there are many kinds of other pain, and the method of pain control will depend on learning just what the cause is. The cancer specialist will probably order a number of tests—X rays, bone scans, CAT scans, etc.—to determine precisely what is causing the pain, because almost 80 percent of the pain problems in cancer occur as acute pain. With proper diagnosis and treatment, there is almost always a dramatic reduction or elimination of the pain.

The greatest number of these acute cancer pain problems— about 50 percent—are due to metastatic bone disease; another 25 percent are the result of tumor compressing or infiltrating nerve; another 3 percent involve tumor of other internal organs.

Nearly 20 percent of cancer pains are actually the result of cancer therapy—surgery or radiation or chemotherapy. For example, patients may receive steroids as part of their chemotherapy. This can lead to loss of calcium from the bones, and a patient may develop a compression fracture of the spine or deterioration of the hip. These conditions can be treated, but obviously the proper diagnosis of the pain is a necessary first step.

Finally, a small percentage of patients may have pain that is not at all related to their cancer or its treatment. After all, cancer patients, like anyone else, can have painful joints or nerve damage or disk problems, etc., and it is important that such pain conditions are properly diagnosed so that they are not confused with the cancer pain, and so that they can be properly treated.

The Use of Analgesics
The greatest difference between the treatment of cancer pain and that of other chronic-pain states is that the cancer pain is treated more like acute pain initially. The underlying cause must be appropriately diagnosed and properly treated. In most cases, the pain then disappears or is brought under adequate control.

But when it is clear that treatment of the underlying cause of the cancer pain does not provide adequate control, then the proper use of analgesics serves as the major part of the pain-control strategy. Like the treatment of acute pain too is the liberal use of analgesics for the control of cancer pain, because there is not the concern for the long-term effects in these cases, as there must be in the other, nonmalignant, chronic-pain conditions.

People whose imaginations cause them to think the worst about cancer pain are usually very surprised to learn that anti-inflammatory drugs, rather than narcotics, are the first line of defense, and aspirin is the most commonly used of this group. Because we can buy this without a prescription, we may think that it could not be very effective. But, just as in the case of rheumatoid arthritis, so in cancer, aspirin is remarkably effective. The International Association for the Study of Pain, in partnership with the World Health Organization, promotes the use of aspirin as the first analgesic for control of cancer pain; it is safe, inexpensive and effective.

The reason for this is that the commonest type of pain in cancer is that involving the bones. This usually causes the production of a chemical called prostaglandin, which is responsible for stimulating the nerve endings that signal pain. Aspirin and the other anti-inflammatory drugs interfere with the production of prostaglandin and so have a specific analgesic effect directly at the site of the injury.

Aspirin and the other anti-inflammatory drugs are nonnarcotic analgesics which are used in the treatment of pain of mild to moderate severity. Unlike narcotics, these drugs, even in long-term use, are not likely to lead to tolerance nor dependence nor addiction. But there is usually a limit to the effectiveness of the anti-inflammatory medications, in that increasing the dose beyond a certain point is of no benefit, and some unpleasant side effects in the stomach and intestines may occur.

If the cancer pain is severe or not adequately controlled with aspirin, then the recommendation is that codeine be added. Codeine is a narcotic analgesic which is most widely used for pain of moderate severity. When combined with an anti-inflammatory analgesic and taken regularly, say, every four hours, to avoid the peaks and valleys of analgesia which we described earlier, this combination will be very effective for the majority of the pains encountered. There are other narcotics of comparable strength to codeine that can be substituted if there are problems with it, just as there are other anti-inflammatory drugs to choose from if there are problems with aspirin. By combining the two types of analgesic, action occurs both at the site of the tumor and in the spinal cord and brain.

The third and final stage of analgesic control occurs when the codeine-aspirin combination (or one comparable to it) proves to be inadequate. In that situation, morphine or one of the other, stronger narcotics is substituted for the codeine. Such drugs can be gradually increased in dosage as necessary to provide very satisfactory pain control. There are several such strong narcotic analgesics to choose from, and when they are used properly, pain can be controlled adequately in almost every case. By this is meant that the pain is either eliminated, or the amount remaining is of no consequence to the patient. There are some exceptions, for which the other methods of pain control are useful.

Judy is 29 years old, is married and has a girl of 5 and a boy who is 3. She is in the hospital with cancer of an ovary which has spread to the liver and other organs. She has been hospitalized both to receive therapy for the cancer and for pain control.

The pain is apparently due both to the mass in her abdomen, which is compressing a number of tissues, and to metastases to the sacral spine and involvement of the nerve roots there. Judy feels the pain as a constant, heavy pressure and "hard ache" in her abdomen, and she considers it to be very severe.

When I see her she is drowsy but uncomfortable. She has been given an intramuscular injection of Demerol, a strong narcotic. Her physician has written orders that she may have this "every four hours *as needed* for pain." This means that Judy can have the injection if she asks for it, but not more frequently than every four hours.

Judy knows she can ask for the injection, but she waits until the pain is very severe before asking, and then the drug makes her so drowsy she can hardly keep awake for the next two hours. She is thus seesawing in the peaks and valleys of not enough and too much analgesia, and her pain is really not very well controlled. In addition, she is obviously very upset about her condition. There are several pictures of her cute little children and her husband on the bedside stand.

At my suggestion, her physician orders codeine and aspirin to be taken orally every three hours; the Demerol injection is kept as a backup if necessary. Judy is also given an antidepressant, which helps her with her emotional control and helps her pain control as well. And we start to talk about her understandable sadness at having to leave her children behind and not seeing them grow up. Within two days Judy's pain is well controlled without the injections, and her inner tension is beginning to lessen. But there is obviously a need for us to keep on talking.

Side Effects
When using narcotics, constipation is almost always a significant problem. This is because there are as many or more opiate receptors in the gut as in the nervous system, and the narcotics work to make the gut stop moving. So as soon as narcotics are prescribed—and for as long as they are taken—the physician will usually prescribe both laxatives and stool softeners so as to avoid this problem.

Some patients may become drowsy when taking narcotics at a strength adequate to provide pain relief. This is sometimes alleviated by taking a slightly smaller amount more frequently, such as every three hours instead of every four.

Usually this problem does not arise when other sedating medications are not also being taken. As old-time pharmacists used to say, "Pain uses up the narcotics." In any event, the physician can usually adjust the dosage so that the sleepiness is brought under control.

Some patients may experience nausea with the narcotic prescribed. This seems to be very variable from one individual to another, and for any individual from one drug to another. If this is a problem, it can usually be alleviated by a change to another narcotic. In some cases, the use of medication to control nausea may be necessary.

Alternative Methods of Pain Control

We have already mentioned that, in the early stages of cancer, the likelihood of pain being a serious problem is very small. The probability of pain occurring increases as the disease progresses. When the pain does occur it requires evaluation, and if the underlying cause is treated appropriately, the pain usually responds as well. It is the resistant pain which is then brought under control with analgesics. But there are a number of other pain-control methods available—already described in this book—which can be used either instead of, or in addition to, the analgesics.

The choice of which technique is most appropriate depends upon the type of pain and how far along in the course of the disease the patient is.

If the pain is generalized in the abdomen but not very severe, then it is probably wisest to begin with mental techniques for pain control. Assuming that chemotherapy and/or radiation have not helped, and cancer surgery is not possible, then mental control is certainly the simplest and safest, and without any significant side effects. Hypnosis, to produce hypnotic analgesia, and teaching the patient self-hypnosis may be all that is necessary. Or visual imagery or other techniques for putting the pain in the background may be used, as well as techniques for pacing activities and the other methods we have already described for pain management.

The first cancer patient with whom I worked for pain control, years ago, was Joe. He was a black-bearded 37-year-old artist, who had cancer of the pancreas. The cancer was resistant to therapy, and Joe was tolerant to high doses of morphine. When I first saw him, he was sweating and restless with pain. He and his wife were part of the counterculture and told me that they were really interested in nontraditional, "alternative" methods of pain control. They had practiced various kinds of meditation and believed in the healing powers of the mind.

We started using hypnosis for pain control. I made a hypnosis tape for Joe to practice with, and he found it very helpful. He said his pain seemed less severe, although it was still there. Then we started using hypnosis to promote the healing of his body and the union of his thoughts with the universal soul. Immediately the tension seemed to leave him, and Joe relaxed and smiled for the first time in weeks. He didn't mention pain again, nor did he ask for any more morphine. He died quietly in his sleep about three weeks later.

If the patient does well with these alternate techniques, he or she may avoid the side effects and complications of analgesics, of nerve blocks and of surgery for pain relief, or at least may be able to postpone these measures until later in the course of the illness. If these mental techniques are not helpful, little has been lost, little time spent, and the other approaches can then be tried.

TENS should be remembered as a pain-control technique. It has been found to be exceptionally effective in certain well-localized cancer pains, such as compression fractures of the spine, or metastases to or pathological fractures of the ribs. It is often also helpful in other pains which arise in the wake of cancer, such as neuropathies (nerve damage) and the neuralgia accompanying or remaining after shingles.

In the advanced and terminal stages of cancer, if pain becomes more severe and cannot be properly controlled with analgesics, then it is entirely appropriate to consider surgery or nerve blocks. The nerve blocks are usually performed by anesthesiologists who have a special interest in and background in the technique. There are certain blocks that are used more commonly than others. For example, an injection into the abdominal nerve center, the celiac plexus, is often used to block the pain of cancer of the pancreas; the pain relief can last for months. Similar blocks are used for pains of the head and neck and of the pelvis or rectum.

Other pain can be controlled by neurosurgical procedures. Depending on the site of the pain, the nerve pathways in the spinal cord may be cut (cordotomy), or part of the spinal cord may be split lengthwise (myelotomy). Such surgery also can provide months of pain relief. There is often some muscle weakness or incoordination which accompanies the loss of sensation from the involved area, but in advanced stages of the disease this is usually felt to be an acceptable price to pay. Other surgical procedures include implanting a reservoir or pump which drips an analgesic like morphine directly onto the spinal cord, and—in a few pain treatment centers—stimulating electrodes may be implanted on the spinal cord or in the brain to block the pain.

Thus, as with the use of analgesics, there are pain-control methods available for cancer pain, especially in the later stages, that would not be used for the other kinds of chronic pain, which are stable rather than progressive. This is because the complications and risks of drug use, nerve blocks and surgery can cause serious problems, and without giving pain relief indefinitely. This is almost always not acceptable in the chronic-pain states, nor early in the course of a malignant disease, but it is perfectly acceptable in the later stages, when comfort is the primary goal for the short span of life remaining.

But I should stress that the use of these nerve-block and neurosurgical techniques is needed only for a small minority of those with cancer. The great majority of patients, even those whose disease is far advanced, can be kept quite comfortable with medication alone, with analgesics, sometimes assisted by antidepressants, which seem to make the analgesics more effective. All the experts who specialize in looking after cancer patients' pain problems seem to agree on this point.

Differences in Attitudes

Most of those who receive the news that they have cancer do so in the early stages of the disease. They are able to go on with their usual lifestyle for quite a while, but obviously must go through a lot of mental adjustments and emotional upheavals as they come to terms with the facts of their illness and its many implications. It is in this adjustment that the great difference exists between those who have cancer pain and those who have other chronic pain.

Hospice care has alerted many people to the need to be sensitive to the emotions and attitudes of those with cancer, and the principles of hospice care are now practiced in many hospitals. Those who have cancer pain are usually relatively far along in their illness, and they must deal with the fact of their *dying*—of which the pain is a constant reminder. Those with other chronic pain must deal with going on *living*, despite the constant pain. There is a basic difference in the kind of problem involved, and so of course there are differences in philosophical outlook and attitudes between the two groups. Those who must learn to live well despite chronic pain need to develop an attitude of determination, sometimes fierce determination, to overcome the pain. Those who must cope with their dying need to develop their acceptance of the fact, gradually surrendering the daily struggle of unessential chores to focus on meaningful relationships and important feelings.

It is very helpful for cancer patients to go on living as usual for as long as they can, but from time to time some adjustments must be made. With cancer patients, as with those whose pain is chronic but stable, there may be a connection between attitude and the severity of the pain.

I have known cancer patients with pain that would not respond to the usual treatments while they struggled to maintain their usual lifestyle and attitudes. But when finally they accepted their dying, seeming to relax inwardly, the pain became easily manageable. It was as though they had focused on the pain as if it were the cause of their difficulties and so blew it up out of proportion to its physical basis.

10.
The Role
of the Family

As difficult and as trying as chronic pain is to the individual, it is every bit as troubling to the family. By "family" I mean all the members of the immediate household, whether related or not, who live together and have regular interactions. Usually they are members of the immediate family, but, for purposes of our discussion here, the actual blood relationship is less important than the proximity and day-to-day dealings with each other.

It is very distressing to see someone you care about in pain, and doubly so if you cannot do anything to help. It is your natural impulse to try to help, to do anything and everything you can to relieve the pain, or at least to offer some comfort. To show your concern, you ask how he or she is feeling. You suggest the person lie down and take it easy, offer to bring the pain pills or the heating pad, or to call the doctor when the pain is especially bad. You feel so frustrated and helpless when nothing that you do or say seems to help. And when the suffering stretches on for months and years, you feel almost as tired and worn out as the person who has the pain.

You've gone to doctor after doctor together, you've spent hours in hospital lobbies and waiting areas, and made countless stops at the pharmacy for dozens of prescriptions at alarming prices. You've had to make night and weekend trips to the emergency room for injections which only bring relief for a few hours. You spend hours every month helping to fill out insurance forms and sweating over your budget because the insurance covers only a fraction of the bills. And all you get for all this effort and worry is *nothing*—no improvement in your loved one's pain, no answers from the doctors, no one seeming to care very much and no end in sight.

In fact it's worse than nothing—the person in pain is more and more cranky, more unpleasant to be around. You never get to do things together anymore, you have more work to do than ever before, you're more giving and more drained than you have ever been and yet you get less back for yourself than ever. There are times you wonder how long you can take it, whether it is worth it. You wish the person in pain could just learn to overcome it somehow. There are times that you feel some resentment over your situation, resentment toward the pain, the doctors, the whole situation, even toward that irritable person in pain. You know it's not his or her fault, it can't be helped, but still you feel the resentment sometimes, and then you feel guilty about feeling that way.

As time goes on, you begin to wonder how you're supposed to act. Are you supposed to give all the help and support you can? Should you give sympathy and tender loving care, or is that "catering to the pain?" Should you ignore the pain and insist that the person act normally, or is that too coldhearted and unsympathetic? Part of the uncertainty comes from your feeling that things could be made to go more smoothly despite the pain, but you're not sure just how you're supposed to go about it.

Part of the problem too is that when something as disruptive as chronic pain occurs in a family, all the usual patterns of relating to one another are disturbed. It is entirely appropriate to treat someone with acute pain with sympathy and tender loving care. But when months go by and the pain becomes chronic, then normal relationships need to be restored. The emergency is over, and now it is time to pick up the pieces and carry on. If not, certain destructive patterns begin to emerge which we can call "pain games."

Family Pain Games

Some pain patients and their families (or friends) play "games" with each other without entirely realizing it. They all feel so sincere about their feelings and intentions that they cannot imagine that they are manipulating each other in order to get a certain payoff—which is what the word "game" means here. And yet that is what they are doing to each other.

The Home Tyrant. The pain patient can become a kind of tyrant at home. A tyrant is one who gets his or her way with the aid of a weapon of some kind, and the patient's pain can be a powerful weapon. It can, for example, help him or her to get out of many responsibilities and still save face. For example:

PAIN PATIENT. It's not that I don't want to (put out the trash, have sex, go to work). I just can't.

SPOUSE (or other relation). That's all right, dear. I understand.

The pain serves as an excuse with honor. Anyone who would insist that the patient live up to his or her responsibilities is made to appear unfeeling and cruel. It is rarely discussed that the pain itself is *not* a disability, and that the word "can't" is inaccurate and really means "don't want to."

And the patient doesn't admit that since he or she is going to be in pain whether lying in bed all the time or doing what should normally be done, he or she might as well get on with the business of living. Since the patient doesn't say it, the others don't either.

In addition to getting out of things he or she would rather not do, the patient, by pain behavior, gets others to do things that the patient could easily do. The pained expression on the face, the gasp, moan or tears, bring attention and concern:

PAIN PATIENT. *(through some behavior)* I'm hurting.

SPOUSE. Should I call the doctor (get your pills, take you to the hospital)?

Each of these things offered by the spouse or other relation is obviously something the patient could do without help. So there is something more going on than just a simple request for help. The patient is giving a reminder of being someone who is suffering. By expressing it, even though the expression does not relieve the pain, he or she provokes guilt feelings and sympathy and attention from others.

And the patient gets all these things without having to admit needing or wanting them—after all, he or she did not ask to be in pain, so the tender loving care can be accepted honorably. But there is a price to pay, because this game playing causes two problems.

1. It reinforces the patient's sick role, because the patient surrenders normal responsibilities and continues having others do what the patient can and should do.

2. It puts an added burden on the spouse or other family member, who has to act like a parent to the childish patient and has no one to reciprocate by giving even normal attention.

The wielding of the pain weapon to bring the family under control can apply to the patient's children as well as the spouse. Without actual discipline, the children can be kept in line by the patient expressing pain and producing guilt feelings in them:

PAIN PATIENT. How could you make so much noise? Can't you see how much I'm hurting?

CHILD: I'm sorry I was noisy. I forgot.

In addition, the patient can actually be abusive to the children and blame it on the pain causing so much irritability.

CHILD. I'm sorry I was noisy. I forgot.

PAIN PATIENT. When I get through with you, you'll never forget again.

So the patient tyrannizes those at home by avoiding responsibilities, controlling family members' behavior by manipulating their guilt and getting payoffs while lying around feeling self-pity.

Marcia, who does all her housework despite being in a wheelchair in pain since the plane crash, says, "My family understands my problem but they are not overly protective. The big plus here is that they understand a little grouchiness or that I sometimes have to drop out of certain activities in order to rest. Otherwise they treat me in a normal fashion and expect a normal amount of attention from me."

Note that Marcia is expected to *give* a normal amount of attention to the family and not just *get* it.

The principle to remember when dealing with one in pain is that tender loving care is appropriate and necessary in the acute-pain situation. It is inappropriate and destructive in the chronic situation. As time goes by, as the weeks pass into months and years and it appears that the pain is going to remain, then patient and family must insist on resuming their normal patterns of activities and ways of dealing with each other.

The family should not feel guilty that the patient is suffering pain; it is not their fault. Nor should the family feel responsible for relieving the patient's pain—that is, if it is possible, the doctor's job. Certainly the family members should not feel so guilty that they fail to stand up for their own rights to live partly independent lives.

Obviously the family should not go to the extreme of ignoring the patient, thereby failing to give the emotional support the patient needs to overcome the handicap of pain. They should give normal attention and support for normal, healthy behavior and conversation and simply not react to expressions of pain.

At the other extreme is the situation, which we have described, in which the family become "doormats" to the tyrannical patient. They do so much for him or her that they actually sabotage any possibility the patient may have of rehabilitation. In pain treatment programs the families are shown how to ignore pain behavior, how to change the subject away from pain topics in conversation and how to reinforce normal, healthy behavior of the patient by giving it attention and occasional appropriate praise. Some families need to be shown how to do these things because it doesn't seem natural to them, but others have no difficulty and pick them up quickly as soon as they know it's all right to do so.

Family Sabotage

It is hard for family members to realize that their acts of kindness and expressions of sympathy are actually harmful to the patient whose pain is chronic. Such a person has to learn how to overcome the pain in order to lead a more normal and satisfying life. Continued expressions of sympathy and doing things for the patient that the patient can do for him- or herself have these effects:

1. The patient is reminded of the pain, so that it is magnified in his or her awareness.

2. The patient is kept from functioning normally and so is kept in a disabled state, unable to do the things he or she would normally be able to do despite pain.

Steve, the Green Beret who had too much sympathy from the nurses and volunteers in the hospital, had the same problem of too much sympathy from friends and family at home.

"They gave me all this tea-and-sympathy crap, and I actually had to tell them to knock it off. That stuff's okay when you're first hurt and feeling sorry for yourself. But, after, when you're trying to pull yourself together and adjust and rehabilitate, it's just sabotage."

Without realizing it, and probably with the kindest intentions in the world, the family can play a "game" of sabotage, which is as nasty in its way as is a tyrant game played by a pain patient. There is a payoff, for some families, in being in control, in keeping someone helpless and dependent on them.

PAIN PATIENT. I think I'll try to take a short walk this morning.

SPOUSE (or other relation). Do you think that's wise? Maybe you should just lie down and take it easy.

<humbr> * * *

This type of conversation undermines the patient's self-confidence and attempt to resume normal activity. In some pain clinics, when this sort of thing is observed, the family member is referred to as an "enabler" or a "reinforcer" of the patient's excessive disability. Rather than encouraging the patient to participate in the rehabilitation program and to resume a normal life, the spouse or other relation tries to "defend" the patient:

DOCTOR. We're going to start you on some physical-therapy exercises so you can function better.

SPOUSE. Isn't that risky? It will just make his (her) pain worse and might cause some damage.

This does not "defend," but rather overprotects the patient. It serves to reinforce the patient's anxiety about the pain and what it might mean and makes the patient overly apprehensive about treatment. It also makes the patient overly dependent upon the relation, relying on his or her opinions and accepting his or her decisions.

And that of course is the real reason why the relation behaves this way. It is not normal caring or kindness or concern, but has the payoff of giving the relation power and control over the patient in a skewed family relationship. When there is a consistent and repeated pattern of reinforcing disabled behavior and undermining progress, the "concern" is really sabotage.

The Healthy Family
What's the answer to the question about how you should deal with the pain patient? You have seen that it is not helpful to

allow the patient to dominate the family by fostering the family's guilt, nor is it helpful for the family to dominate the patient by fostering the patient's dependency. These kinds of manipulations may give some kinds of payoff, satisfy some needs, but they are not best for the patient nor for you.

When the pain is new, whether from disease or injury, then of course you give all the attention and sympathy that you can and that the patient needs. But when the pain persists beyond the normal healing time, and when the doctors indicate that it is obvious that the pain is here to stay—certainly after six months or so (to give you a ball-park estimate)—then it is time to start having some discussions all around.

First, you need to know from the doctor what it is safe for the patient to do. If the pain is chronic, then it is no longer a warning signal but just a "false alarm." Does this mean that the pain can safely be ignored and normal activities resumed? Ask the doctor.

Watch out for phrases the doctor may use, like "Let the pain be your guide," or "If it hurts, don't do it." Jump on these immediately and get them clarified. Just what does the doctor mean—that the pain *is* a warning signal of possible damage or harm? If so, what might happen, and what limitations or precautions should be followed? If there is no risk, if the doctor is only referring to keeping a certain comfort level, then that needs to be made clear so that the patient, and the family too, can start gradually increasing activities, using their own judgment as a guide.

Then there needs to be some discussion in the family about how changes are going to be made. Things need to get back to normal, or as nearly so as possible, but obviously not all at once. If the patient has been pretty much out of commission for six months or more, a reasonable time schedule needs to be worked out for the patient to resume gradually his or her normal responsibilities.

You, as family, need to have an attitude of encouraging the patient's improvement. If there is some disability such as muscle weakness or paralysis in addition to the pain, then a complete return to normal may not be possible, but some significant improvement should be. You will be patient as your loved one works toward improvement, using the techniques we have described, but nevertheless you will definitely expect to see progress.

You will always praise progress, give compliments for each small step, give pats on the back and hugs for each improvement and generally give emotional support. But you must make clear to the patient that for his or her own good, you are now going to ignore all the usual pain behaviors—grunts or moans or sighs or limping or clutching the area or facial expressions. The patient now has to start acting normal again and give up the sick role, and all these behaviors are an important part of the identity of an invalid. So the family must stop reinforcing them and ignore them.

You should expect the patient to work at both the physical conditioning and the mental exercises which we have described, and you should know what they are so you can talk about them. If you have the time and the patient is willing, you should do the exercises together. Having company is very helpful and supportive; and the patient will feel as though he or she has a real partner and is not so alone.

But one thing you must not do is nag. Sick and disabled behavior must be ignored, not scolded. You cannot get into a parent-child role, for that skews the healthy relationship into an unhealthy one. If the patient agrees to work on making progress but does not follow through, then you need to have further discussions. Some persons are just unable to get going on their own no matter how much they want to or how hard they try. This may be because of a personality problem or because the pain is so severe or for other reasons.

If you and the patient cannot make a go of the rehabilitation at home under your doctor's guidance, then it's time for another conference. It may be that you'll need to consider a pain treatment center with a strong rehabilitation program. A more closely supervised, systematic program that incorporates many of the principles we have been describing in this book will have an excellent chance of helping the patient to reach the highest level of functioning possible—and thus the most satisfying life possible.

In a nutshell, then, your family attitude should be one of patient, hopeful expectation of progress. And your family behavior should be one of simply not paying attention to or reacting to pain behavior, but giving attention to normal healthy behavior and compliments for all signs of progress.

11.
Dealing with Doctors

If you have chronic pain, you are going to need a special relationship with a special kind of medical doctor. You are going to need to understand the doctor's role, the patient's role and the doctor-patient relationship far better than the average person does. And you will have to watch yourself carefully so that you don't allow your pain to make you say those things or play those "games" that can alienate your doctor.

To begin with, you must understand that most doctors still do not understand how to help a patient manage chronic pain. They are used to thinking of all pain as acute pain, that is, an acute symptom of an underlying disease or injury. There is an almost automatic reflex to order tests to discover the cause of the pain, to reach for the prescription forms to give you some analgesic relief while the studies are being carried out and to expect to be able to provide you with appropriate medical or surgical treatment for the underlying pathology once a diagnosis has been made.

This is entirely correct for acute-pain states and results in success in a very high percentage of cases. But if you have chronic pain, you have almost certainly been through all that, perhaps even several times, and at this point most doctors are likely to feel frustrated that their usual way of proceeding is not effective. So if your doctor, who has coordinated the search for the cause and cure for your pain, bringing in various consultants at times, has not been able to find or correct the underlying problem, he or she is likely to feel at a loss.

If this is the situation, you must not back your doctor into a corner by insisting on getting pain relief. Out of compassion, your doctor may try to help, and then you'll both be sorry— because, as we have seen, the traditional medical and surgical methods for relieving acute and cancer pain usually backfire in treating chronic pain.

Many people in pain think it is the doctor's responsibility to alleviate the pain. Doctors also think so, believing that if they cannot cure, they can at least comfort those who are suffering. But the doctor's primary responsibility is to find and treat the underlying pathology, and the patient has the "obligation" of providing the pathology to treat. If you do not show evidence of such pathology, or if it is not treatable, then you do yourself no good by insisting on relief. You must back off and consider the choices available to you and your doctor for pain relief.

Surgery, not to correct some problem but just to provide pain relief, is helpful in only a few kinds of pain (see Chapter 4). Because there are usually side effects and the pain often returns, surgical pain relief is usually reserved for cases of terminal illness, when the patients are likely to die before the pain recurs.

Prescription analgesics usually lead to the many problems we described in Chapter 8. You would be foolish to insist on your doctor continuing to supply you with these, especially since there are so many effective alternatives that are safer.

Tranquilizers may help if you are very nervous, but they tend to dull and confuse your mind and make you more depressed, and they are definitely habit-forming.

Your doctor may suggest that you see a psychologist or psychiatrist to get help in learning to live with the pain, but the majority of these "shrinks" seldom deal with chronic-pain problems, being more used to treating mental illness and emotional problems. If you do see one, you should try to find one who has worked with a pain treatment center.

What is left? Just two things. You can decide to make it on your own, following the steps outlined in this book. Or, if you feel you cannot do this, you can ask your doctor to refer you to one of the specialized pain treatment centers around the country.

But let's look now at the relationship between you and your doctor. There are, first of all, certain things you should not do, in addition to not insisting that he or she provide you with pain relief. These are things that spoil an honest and open and helpful relationship.

Pain Games
Just as in the family relationship, which we described in the previous chapter, pain can be used to manipulate the other party in order to obtain a certain benefit or payoff. But people, including doctors, do not like to be manipulated; they feel used and tricked. Here are some of the commonest pain games that chronic-pain patients use with doctors, and which you need to be wary of in yourself.

The Professional. The "professional patient," like the professional athlete, is one who is paid for his role. You lose your amateur (acute patient) standing when you accept financial reward for being a pain patient. This may come in the form of compensation claims, litigation suits, unemployment benefits, welfare payments, social security disability benefits, etc.

The problem is that you need to have your doctor certify you as disabled, even though pain alone is not a disability. So you have to run a game on the doctor in which at first you don't ask for disability or whatever, but ask for pain relief instead. You know that relief is impossible, or at least that nothing works completely, still you insist that the doctor do something to take away your pain. Then, because of feeling guilty for failing, the doctor will be more likely to agree to some kind of financial reward for you. The outline of the game goes like this:

PAIN PATIENT. Please fix me (but you'll fail).

DOCTOR. I'll fix you.

PAIN PATIENT. How long before I can go back to work?

DOCTOR. Not just yet—we'll see.

PAIN PATIENT. Sign here.

The point is that you can't appear to want to avoid work. In fact, you have to act as if the thing you want most in the world is to return to work and you are impatient with the doctor for restraining you. This applies even if you have not worked for a number of years and realistically cannot return to your former job because someone else has it now and you are not physically able anyway. You also brush aside any suggestion that you consider another kind of work. You insist on wanting your usual work, and you consider yourself disabled if you cannot perform your old job.

Now, in fact, we know that very few pain patients are totally disabled. Almost everyone can do something. It is not your doctor's job to find an alternative career for you—that is your responsibility. If your doctor is alert to what you are doing and is really interested in doing what is best for you despite your game, he or she will do something like this:

PAIN PATIENT. Sign here.

DOCTOR. O.K. I'm writing here that this is for three months only. By that time, I'm sure you'll have found some other kind of work you can do despite your pain. You're not totally disabled, you know.

The reason why it is important that you *not* be a "professional pain patient" is that you could not afford to get better if your income depended on your having pain and disability. It is a common observation from pain programs around the country that those patients who have litigation pending, or who have disability incomes because of their pain, have poor outcomes from treatment. In fact, many pain treatment centers refuse to take such patients any longer, because it is such a waste of time. Those who have a financial incentive or financial reward for their pain simply do not show any motivation to improve, despite ample evidence from their evaluations that they could improve significantly. The price to be paid for such refusal to make progress, however, is continued excessive pain and excessive disability.

The Addict. Very few pain patients admit to their need for narcotic analgesics. In fact, you probably dislike taking drugs. But you may be frightened by your pain, and during the acute stage of the pain problem you learned that narcotics would control the pain. Several analgesics were tried, and you learned which one worked best. But it's usually the strongest, and the doctors usually are nervous about continuing to prescribe it, and so you are stuck with a weak analgesic that hardly works at all. You must maneuver the doctor into prescribing the strong one again:

PAIN PATIENT. When the pain came on last night, I took the Darvon you gave me, and it didn't work, so I took some Talwin my neighbor had and some codeine that Doctor Pushover had prescribed for me, and it only eased the pain a little bit. I hate taking all those pills. Can't you cut a nerve or something instead?

DOCTOR. I wish we could, but let's find a more effective analgesic since the others aren't helping you. You won't become addicted if you follow directions.

Now that the right drug is prescribed—and it may take a few trials—it is necessary to ensure a steady supply. As with the litigation or compensation or disability claim, it is important not to appear as if you want it. (This is like the old Uncle Remus tale of Brer Rabbit pleading with Brer Fox *not* to throw him in the briar patch—which is just where he wants to go.)

PAIN PATIENT. Doctor, this pain is excruciating. It's driving me out of my mind. Isn't there something you can do?

DOCTOR. Do you mean the pain's worse?

PAIN PATIENT. No, it's better controlled now with that Percodan you prescribed, it at least takes the edge off. But I hate to take drugs like this. Can't you operate?

DOCTOR. (*relieved*) No, I think we'd better just keep things as they are for now.

If this sort of thing has happened with you, then you are headed for all the analgesic problems we described in Chapter

8—tolerance, dependence and addiction, plus the probable long-term complications of kidney and possibly liver problems. If your doctor is aware of the issues and can stand firm against your manipulations in order to do what is best for you, then something like this will take place:

PAIN PATIENT. I hate taking all those pills. Can't you cut a nerve or something instead?

DOCTOR. I think you're right about those pills. They don't seem to help, and they'll only mess you up. Stop taking them.

PAIN PATIENT. But what about the pain? It's driving me crazy, it's unbearable.

DOCTOR. You're just going to have to live with it. There are safer ways of managing it than drugs. If you can't overcome the pain on your own, we can find a good pain treatment center for you.

If you have chronic pain that is not associated with a terminal disease, you know now that drugs are not a good answer for long-term pain control. They are wonderful for short-term, acute pain and for pain of advanced terminal disease, but the alternative strategies we have described in this book are more effective for chronic, nonmalignant pain.

The Confounder. For some patients the payoff of their game with doctors seems to be one of winning "stump the doctor." When they developed their pain problem, they made the rounds of a number of doctors, hospitals and even pain clinics, becoming angrier and more bitter as they failed to get the relief they wanted. So they just continue on these rounds, telling themselves that they are just trying to get help but actually getting a kind of revenge on doctors by getting them to promise help and then showing the doctors up.

The way to do this is to start having a good response to whatever is tried by the doctor. That draws the doctor into the trap, and then you can spring it and "stump the chump." Every pain treatment program has had at least one patient do something like this:

PAIN PATIENT. I'm sure happy to be accepted here, Doctor. This is the best program I've ever seen. The other patients tell me how much you've helped them, and I'm beginning to feel really hopeful. You people sure know what you're doing.

DOCTOR. (*embarrassed*) I'm glad of that, and I hope we'll help you too.

PAIN PATIENT. (*three weeks later*) Doctor, this program is terrific. I haven't felt this good in years. I don't know how to thank you.

DOCTOR. (*pleased*) That's very good news, thank you.

PAIN PATIENT. (*two months later, tearfully*) Doctor, the pain is back and it's worse than ever. What did you do?

DOCTOR. (*frustrated*) I don't understand. We'll have to look at you again.

With the history from the patient's old records, it should have been obvious what was happening. With every admission or every treatment there was an initial favorable response, followed by a dramatic worsening.

The only way that this game can be stopped is by predicting that it will happen. That makes the doctor seem like he or she is the winner of the game, rather than the loser. Because if the pain returns "worse than ever," then the patient has proved the doctor was right. But if the patient improves and stays better, then the doctor looks like the winner!

PAIN PATIENT. I'm beginning to feel really hopeful. You people sure know what you're doing.

DOCTOR. Thanks, but I'm not hopeful at all. In fact, I'm very pessimistic, to be frank with you. If you do get better it will be due more to your willpower than to anything we can do. If you don't get better, I won't be surprised, considering your history.

PAIN PATIENT. *(three weeks later)* I don't know how to thank you.

DOCTOR. Don't thank us, what did we do? You helped yourself. And we'll see if it lasts. Don't forget, your pain has always gotten worse after treatment in the past. Whether it remains improved now is entirely up to you. I'm skeptical, but we'll see.

Obviously, all these games are really silly and self-defeating. Probably no more than 10 percent of pain patients play some version of a pain game very seriously. The reason for including these examples here is chiefly to alert you to the kind of trap you might fall into if you aren't careful. The games involve manipulation of another for the sake of a pay-off. It usually results in considerable irritation or resentment on the part of the one who was conned. Since you are going to have your pain for a long time, and you need a good relationship with your doctor for a long time as well, it doesn't make sense to win some short-term gain but lose a good long-term relationship which depends on mutual trust.

The Better Relationship

You have an important problem simply trying to find a doctor who is willing to manage your care. Many doctors don't like to work with chronic-pain patients any more than mechanics like to work on cars that are "lemons." Patients with chronic pain tend to be angry and demanding and never satisfied, because they cannot get better. They are not really sick enough to treat, they have a problem that can't be solved, they come in with long lists of symptoms and complaints like hypochondriacs, and they're likely to be just a royal pain in the neck. That's how many doctors see chronic-pain patients, and although it is part of our tendency to "blame the victim," you might as well be aware of it.

So if and when you find a physician who is willing to manage and coordinate your care, you would be wise to treat the relationship respectfully. You and your doctor should spell out to each other what you expect, what is reasonable. The relationship of doctor and chronic-pain patient is a little different from the usual doctor-patient relationship because your needs are a little different. We could list a great number of topics that you might want to discuss with your physician, but these are very variable from one patient to another, so we will consider just a few points relative to chronic pain generally.

You and your doctor have a right to expect certain things from one another. For example, you should be able to have a periodic (once or twice a year) reevaluation of your pain problem to see if it is progressive or if any significant change has occurred, without being made to feel like a hypochondriac. But your doctor should be able to examine you without having to wade through a volume of your notes and diaries describing every possible physical symptom and body sensation. If you don't act like a hypochondriac, you probably won't be treated like one. If you feel as though you are being treated like a hypochondriac, you need to discuss that, to find out if it's something you are doing or saying. If it is not, then it's fair to ask the doctor to stop making you feel that way.

Your doctor should feel free of pressure from you to "do something" about the pain when you both know that nothing more can be done. If he or she feels pressure from you, it implies that you feel your doctor is incompetent unless you are provided with more relief. When pain is chronic, it is really up to you to overcome it, using the methods of physical and mental pain control we have described.

Similarly, there should not be any "emergency" phone calls about your chronic pain—nothing chronic, not even chronic pain, is an emergency. On the other hand, a new pain, or a dramatic change in your usual pain, may indeed be an emergency, and you should be able to report it to your doctor without fear of being made to feel like a hypochondriac. If you have not abused your reporting of the usual chronic pain, like the boy who cried, "Wolf!" in *Aesop's Fables*, then you'll get a respectful hearing when you do have something new and different to report.

You should be able to learn from your doctor when new developments arise in pain research or techniques of pain treatment. You should not have to shop around to find the best relief available, or pry information from your doctor. On the other hand, not everything that is written up in newspapers and magazines or reported on television is really proved and ready for use. Your doctor keeps up with the medical journals and required continuing medical education courses, and it's enough if he or she keeps eyes and ears open. You should spare your doctor from a bombardment of questions about everything you notice in the media.

Your doctor should be able to count on you to be responsible for your own life. It is not your doctor's responsibility to find you a job, rehabilitate you or solve your family problems. But if your doctor thinks you are becoming too depressed or withdrawn or irritable, he or she should be able to refer you to a psychologist or psychiatrist without your acting insulted about it.

We could continue with a list of examples like this, but by now you get the idea. These mutual expectations must be appropriate and not unreasonable. When you are always hurting, it is natural that from time to time you may regress to a childish stage emotionally and want to make unreasonable demands on the doctor. You may want to act toward the doctor much the way a child does toward its mother or father, either pleading for help or angrily demanding it. These reactions are not only natural but understandable, but you really cannot allow them to put the doctor on the spot, especially when there is no further help to be given.

All of this boils down to two basic points. First, you and your doctor must have good communications so that you feel free to be open with each other and to talk frankly without becoming too emotional. And second, you must be fair with each other so that neither you nor your doctor make unreasonable demands on the other.

12.
Reasons for Hope

The miserable have no other medicine
But only hope.

—*William Shakespeare*

Periodically you may feel discouraged and worn out. The constant nature of the pain seems to exhaust you, draining your energy and your spirits. You are able to cope with your pain most of the time, using the principles described in this book, but no matter what you do, from time to time your pain seems to get you down. It seems as though it is always present and lying in wait for you, and when your resistance is lowered for a moment, when you let your guard down, the pain overwhelms you.

This may occur at night, when your pain awakens you and you can't get back to sleep, and you are feeling very tired and (understandably) very sorry for yourself. Or you may get up feeling this way some morning, and the feeling of discouragement and even despair may last throughout the day or for several days. You may begin to wonder how long you can go on, or even whether you want to try to go on. Your thoughts sink as low as your mood. You may begin to be very frightened by your thoughts, and a scared feeling is added to your feeling of deep despair.

If you feel this way from time to time, you are not alone. Many persons with chronic pain report the same thing. Every once in a while, a feeling like this comes over them and is hard to shake. The thing that helps seems to be the awareness that this feeling is temporary and will pass. It always does.

You need to treat this bleak mood just as you do flare-ups of severe pain—move your muscles and change your thoughts. Talk to someone, force yourself into some activity, get physically and mentally involved in something different, and the bad spell can be broken. Allowing yourself to dwell on the morbid thoughts can make you feel as if you are going to drown in deep depression. You do not need to let this happen. As soon as you realize that you are in a bad mental and emotional state because of your pain, you should:

- remember that this is a natural but temporary reaction, and it will pass;
- remember that there are reasons to be optimistic, reasons not to give up hope (we describe some of these below);
- immediately get up and change what you are doing, get involved in doing something different physically, which also occupies your thoughts (see the section on Emergency Actions at the end of Chapter 6).

There *are* reasons to remain hopeful. There are new developments in pain research that give us all reasons for hope. These advances are taking place in the fields of neurophysiology, neurochemistry, psychology, pharmacology and neurobiology. Rather than attempt to describe the technical research occurring in these areas, I will use the same categories of applied areas of pain control that we used in Chapter 4. The descriptions in that chapter were a brief outline of the main strengths and limitations of various pain-control methods. In this chapter, however, we will give brief descriptions of what may lie in the future for these methods. This is based on trends in current research, which give an indication of things to come.

Progress in research is never steady. There are usually periods of sudden breakthroughs and insights, alternating with slower periods of filling in the details. There was a period of very rapid growth in pain neurophysiology which began about 1965 and continued for about ten years. Then a comparable period of growth in pain neurochemistry began in 1975 and has continued for about the same length of time. We may expect comparable advances in other fields to occur soon.

Let us look ahead now to some of the reasons for remaining hopeful.

Surgery

Clinical experience with past attempts to control pain by destroying nerves or nerve pathways has been—with a few exceptions—disappointing. Sometimes there would be no relief at all, and other times there would be initial relief but a slow, gradual return of pain, often worse in kind and severity.

The exceptions have been noteworthy, however. In trigeminal neuralgia, which involves recurrent, lightninglike pain of the head or face, neurosurgeons have been able to make radio-frequency lesions in the nerve center, the trigeminal ganglion, which eliminates the pain in a very high percentage of cases.

Recently there have been two new developments related to this problem. One has involved simply bathing the nerve center in glycerol, an oily liquid, which seems to desensitize the ganglion and which has a similar success rate without destroying any nerve cells. And there now is strong evidence that the problem often is caused by a small blood vessel sagging onto the trigeminal nerve root. Putting a small pad between the arteriole and the nerve root can also eliminate pain without destroying tissue.

In the pain of causalgia, a burning pain usually in an arm or leg and due to partial destruction of sympathetic nerve fibers, neurosurgeons have long been able to provide relief by completely cutting the nerves—a sympathectomy—*if* this was done soon after the injury. Now, there has also been demonstrated a relatively effective neurosurgical procedure for relieving arm pain due to damage to the nerves as they enter the spinal cord. It is a technique for making small radio-frequency lesions in the back of the cord, from where the damaged nerve cells have been sending injury signals to the brain.

Since neurosurgeons have adopted the technique of using operating microscopes during surgery and have applied research laboratories' new discoveries of pain pathways, there is an increasing interest in developing new surgical methods for pain control. More and more, we are seeing new techniques tried for different types of chronic pain, and undoubtedly some will prove quite successful and will become standard methods for pain control.

Aside from the approach of finding and destroying damaged nerve cells that fire off indiscriminate pain signals, neurosurgeons have explored the implantation of several kinds of electrical stimulators (see p. 203), as well as reservoirs and pumps for releasing small amounts of analgesics directly into nerve centers and pathways to block pain signals. This last is currently used chiefly for terminal patients, but we may hope to see refinements and improvements in the technique and the development of new anesthetics, which may make this approach useful for other kinds of chronic pain as well.

In most areas of science and medicine, great advances have followed new developments in technology—new instruments which make possible a different way of looking at or doing things. Currently there is a great deal of interest and excitement among surgeons because of new imaging methods, which are used by radiologists for visualizing various structures within the body. It is now possible to use different kinds of scanners to see within the body, and to do so with a precision so astonishing that very small lesions within the nervous system can be detected. This is giving neurosurgeons the opportunity to change their views about whether and how it might be possible to correct some of the defects that account for some chronic-pain problems.

We cannot say that all chronic pain will someday be relieved surgically, but it is certainly true that in the last few years more types of pain have been shown to have a surgical solution, and there is good reason to expect that some other kinds will, too, as great advances are being made.

Nerve Blocks

Anesthesiologists who have a special interest in producing regional anesthesia (nerve blocks which deaden sensations in a part of the body) have also benefited from the new radiological imaging techniques. They can better visualize the structures they are concerned with and better plan and observe their needle placement.

For many years now it has been possible to provide temporary nerve blocks in various parts of the body, much as dentists do while doing some dental procedures. A series of sympathetic nerve blocks done soon after injury can very often prevent or reverse the development of causalgia. Pelvic and abdominal and neck and head pains due to cancer can be relieved by "permanent" nerve blocks, which last long enough to give the patient relief until death. But there is reason to think that it may be possible to use different chemicals than the traditional toxic alcohol and phenol, which were meant to deaden nerve fibers. Since the successful neurosurgical use of glycerol to desensitize the trigeminal nerve, there have been some attempts to use a similar approach for other types of chronic pain.

The use of nerve blocks has an advantage over surgical approaches in that incisions are not necessary. It is only necessary to place a needle tip in the right place, a technique made easier by the new visualizing methods. With the development of new chemicals for desensitizing nerve fibers and bundles of fibers, one can imagine the possibility of being able to control pain in various parts of the body for months at a time. When the effect wears off, it would then be possible to have a repeat injection. It may be possible for some patients to have pain control by means of getting a nerve block about two or three times a year. This is not now a reality, but it is theoretically possible and may yet come to pass.

Electrical Stimulation

In the early 1970s, there was a wave of enthusiasm for the use of dorsal-column stimulators, electrical devices implanted on the spinal cord, for blocking pain signals. There were some very dramatic cases of pain relief, and initial success rates were quite high, but then there was a high rate of failure as time went on. In follow-up studies, long-term good pain control was achieved in only a very small percentage of cases.

The placing of stimulating electrodes in the brain and around big peripheral nerve bundles has also had a good initial success and subsequent high failure rate, although far fewer patients were involved than in neurosurgical attempts at pain control using dorsal-stimulator implants. The same theory lay behind all these approaches: rather than trying to destroy tissue, modulate the activity in the nervous system instead, so as to block the pain signals in a more natural way.

Because of the high failure rate of these early studies, the use of electrical stimulation fell out of fashion. It is now being done in only a few pain treatment and research centers. But in these centers it is recognized that many of the early failures were due to technical equipment failures: slipping of the electrodes, wires breaking, failure of implanted antennae, etc. And just as there have been great advances in the technology of cardiac pacemakers, so there have been significant improvements in these "nerve pacemakers," or implanted neurostimulators.

We can expect to see continued development and improvement of techniques and devices for electrical stimulation, and then neurosurgeons will use them more widely and with greater success than in the past. There is a great deal of research going on in the whole area of "electrical medicine," which will undoubtedly benefit the field of pain control. We have already seen many technical improvements in the externally applied transcutaneous electrical nerve stimulators (TENS), and expect that those who cannot get adequate relief with TENS may yet hope that future advances in implanted stimulators will be helpful.

Chemical Pain Control

Of all the areas of pain research, that of neurochemistry (and neuropharmacology) is currently the most promising. There has been a great deal of intriguing research lately, especially in two areas: opiate receptors and neurotransmitters, called peptides. The results of these studies are very exciting.

Opiate receptors are very small sites on the surface of nerve cells that respond to circulating molecules of narcotics. When the narcotic molecule fits into the opiate receptor, the nerve cell reacts by becoming relatively insensitive to incoming injury signals. There are nerve cells with opiate receptors throughout the brain and spinal cord (and in the intestines, too, which accounts for the side effect of constipation when opiates are taken). The opiate receptors have been known to exist for many years, but it has only been recently that their shapes and sensitivity have begun to be defined.

It turns out that there are several kinds of opiate receptors. Only one of them, the mu receptor, has its primary sensitivity to the narcotic drugs that are in current use. That means that there are three or four opiate receptors, at least, whose chemical keys are still to be clarified. In some preliminary laboratory experiments, these chemicals have shown the promise of being different kinds of analgesics altogether. Many researchers believe that those who have developed a tolerance to one class of narcotic drugs will not be tolerant to drugs of another class.

There is a great deal of interest in this area now because of the possibility of discovering new kinds of analgesics which may not have the drawbacks of the current group of narcotics. We described some of the problems with narcotics in Chapter 8. These include the development of tolerance, dependence and addiction—three different but equally serious problems, which accompany continued use of the drugs—as well as complicating side effects, such as constipation and the suppression of respiration and the cough reflex.

Because of the possibility of great sales if a new and effective analgesic could be developed without one or more of these drawbacks, it is not hard to imagine the pharmaceutical companies putting a lot of effort into research and development of totally new analgesics. Thus there is every reason to expect some breakthroughs in this area in the next few years.

The peptides are another interesting story. They are chemicals that function as neurotransmitters, that is, they are the means by which one nerve cell triggers the next one, the mechanism of communication between nerve cells. Some peptides are involved as messengers in the transmission of injury (pain) signals and others in the transmission of analgesic (pain-inhibiting) signals. Several of this latter group have been analyzed, and the enkephalins particularly seem to have an important analgesic role. There are two of these, l-enkephalin (leucine-enkephalin) and met-enkephalin (methionine-enkephalin), which seem particularly important, and met-enkephalin especially seems to be essential for analgesia.

It is naturally of interest to learn whether artificial or synthetic met-enkephalin, or one of the other peptides, will have possibilities as a totally different, nonopiate analgesic. There are ways of changing their chemical structure so that their action lasts for hours, instead of a fraction of a second. If this is done, and early laboratory studies show that the altered peptides have analgesic effects, then the way may be open to clinical trials of promising nonnarcotic analgesics.

Related to these peptides are some chemicals in the brain known as amines. Of these, serotonin and dopamine seem to function as neurotransmitters in different branches of the descending pain-inhibitory system. In some clinical studies, antidepressant drugs which act on nerve cells containing serotonin have been shown to have analgesic effects in pain patients quite independent of their antidepressant effects. This naturally leads to speculation that drugs designed to have a special effect on one or another of these brain amines may prove to be useful as analgesics in their own right or as boosters to one of the new class of analgesics being developed.

All in all, this is an exciting time of discovery in neuropharmacology and neurochemistry. There is a feeling of optimism that careful and patient work will result in the development of new kinds of chemicals that will be efective in controlling pain, but without the drawbacks and side effects of the present group of narcotic analgesics.

Body Treatments

There are many ways of manipulating and stimulating the body by hand in order to relieve pain. There are chiropractic manipulations, Rolfing, Swedish and various other kinds of massage techniques, shiatsu, or acupressure, and others. Each has its special approach and theory, and each claims special benefits for its technique, but there is no systematic research being done to advance knowledge in the field or to test the different ideas offered. It is unlikely that there will be any breakthroughs. But the stimulation of muscles and other soft tissues is comforting and relaxing, and some pain patients feel that, even though there is no long-term benefit, it is worthwhile to get some brief and temporary slight reduction in their pain from time to time.

Psychological Approaches

In the past ten or fifteen years, the several psychological techniques we described in Chapter 6 have been applied in a more refined and systematic way to the management of pain. Previously available only as isolated methods, they have been assembled by psychologists into a well-organized training program, which is now a part of most pain treatment programs in one form or another. So successful has this been that the approach has now been adapted to the needs of behavioral medicine centers, which train people in stress reduction, weight loss, eradication of eating disorders or smoking and modification of other health-related behaviors.

At first, the emphasis was on changing behaviors, getting pain patients over their invalidism and into more healthy behavior patterns. The technique of operant conditioning, the reward system we described in an earlier chapter, was used. This produced good results, but some psychologists then added training in the various mental (cognitive) techniques of pain control, and these are receiving increasing attention in pain centers and being incorporated into the training programs. When Marcia said, "When the pain is bad, I rise above it. It's a mental thing. The higher the pain goes, the higher my mind goes to surmount it," she was describing a kind of self-hypnosis or cognitive technique. She learned it by herself, but other patients can be taught to do it.

There is now interest in research to discover which of the several behavioral and cognitive techniques is most effective for which kinds of patients and for which kind of pain problem. At present, most pain treatment programs use a variety of approaches on all patients, and although overall results are quite good, it is not possible to say which of the program elements is responsible for the improvements observed. So there are plans to do research in which first one treatment, then another, is tried on certain kinds of pain problems to see which is most effective. It is of some interest, because if this research can be done, then treatments can be tailored more exactly to the needs of each patient, and more effective results can be obtained.

There is a widespread belief that our minds have potentials which we have left largely untapped. Researchers in cognitive sciences are exploring mental functions in a systematic way, studying how we think, how we remember, how we solve problems, how we control our body functions, etc. This represents the first time that there has been a very widespread and systematic study of how the mind works, and old ways of thinking about the mind—thinking about thinking—are changing dramatically. It is possible that this research as well will lead to improved techniques for acquiring better mental control of pain.

*　　*　　*

What we have described in this chapter are some of the areas in which pain research is moving forward. Naturally we cannot promise that there will be any dramatic cure for chronic pain, or even that there will be a major breakthrough in any of these areas. Obviously, there cannot be any guarantees. But it is true that there is certainly reason to be optimistic that there will be continued improvement in our knowledge and understanding of pain mechanisms and in our ability to control pain. There are more and more researchers doing basic research in laboratory studies of pain, and there are more and more who are doing systematic clinical research as well. We still need more funding and support for pain research, both by the federal government and by private foundations, but it seems that there is now a momentum which is very encouraging.

Because the problem of pain crosses many disease categories, those who do pain research come from many different medical and psychological specialties and research disciplines. They have different scientific backgrounds and orientations. Thus, at meetings of the International Association for the Study of Pain (IASP) and of the American Pain Society and the other national chapters of the IASP, there is a feeling of excitement as scientists with these different backgrounds and ways of thinking about pain share their ideas and latest research findings. The journal *Pain* is taken at all the medical schools and medical libraries around the world and is referenced in the major listings of medical and scientific research, so researchers of any background can easily consult the articles published in it.

The effect of all this is to make more scientists aware of developments in the field, and more doctors too are becoming aware of the latest ways of treating and of thinking about pain, its mechanisms and its control. More young people are becoming interested in pain as a problem and in doing research on it. As they get involved in the process, they introduce new ways of thinking about problems, some of which lead to different lines of research.

Once again, the entire field of pain research is growing very rapidly, and significant progress is being made. So you can be sure that, no matter how discouraged you may get from time to time, you really have every reason to remain hopeful.

13.
Steps Toward Pain Control—a Summary

The steps listed here are a summary of the principles described in this book. This summary is meant chiefly as a quick review for those who have read this book and wish to refresh their memories, or who wish a convenient checklist to make sure they are making progress in all important areas and are not overlooking something.

These steps summarize the experience of others who have learned to cope, to live well despite pain. You should plan to work on all the steps at the same time. This is not a sequence, in which you work at step one, and when you finish you go on to step two, etc. Rather, each step represents a different area of your life and your pain problem, and you must work at all areas at the same time in order to make progress.

1. *Accept the fact of having chronic pain.*

If you have had appropriate and adequate medical evaluations, and the cause of your chronic pain is understood, and nothing can be done about it, then you must accept the fact that you have this problem and make the best life you can despite it. You should neither give in to pain and just lie around feeling sorry for yourself nor waste your time chasing after some impossible cure. There is much that you can do for yourself, and the more you do, the less pain will dominate your life.

2. Set specific goals for work, recreation or hobbies and social activities toward which you will work.

These goals, things you actually want to accomplish, are those which will keep you busy and bring you satisfaction and occupy your mind. If you want to have a job or need an occupation, then you must work at getting and keeping one. If you do not need an actual paying job, then you should have some worklike activity that gives you a sense of accomplishment, whether as a volunteer or in some other capacity. For fun and a change of pace, you also need some regular hobby or recreational activity. And you need social activities and interaction with family and friends for needed emotional support. You need to be very specific in just exactly what you want to accomplish in these three areas, and you need to work toward these goals in a deliberate, step-by-step manner.

3. Let yourself get angry at your pain if it seems to be getting the best of you.

Do not take your anger and frustrations out on your family or others around you. And do not take it out on yourself, blaming yourself or making yourself depressed. Rather, it is the pain which is the source of your misery, and you should allow yourself to get angry at it and resolve to overcome it. Use your anger at the pain as a source of motivation to pursue the goals you want to accomplish and to use the other steps as a means of achieving these goals. By doing so, you will turn your anger into an effective means of conquering the pain, in that the pain may still be there, but you will have managed to live a satisfying life despite it.

4. *Take your analgesics on a strict time schedule, and then taper off them.*

Long-term use of narcotic analgesics leads to tolerance, physical dependence and addiction, and also has unpleasant side effects. Narcotics taken "as needed" in chronic-pain states tend to have the paradoxical effect of maintaining pain at an abnormally high level, as well as keeping you more mentally dull and irritable than you want to be. Most chronic-pain patients function much better when they withdraw in a gradual and systematic way from narcotics. Nonprescription (over-the-counter) analgesics, when used in large amounts for long periods, can have serious effects on kidneys and liver. If you do not get some pain relief from the small amounts recommended in directions for their use, then stop taking them as well.

5. *Get in the best physical shape possible, then keep fit.*

In order to work at and achieve your goals for work or worklike activity, recreation and social activities, you need to be in sufficiently good condition that pursuing them will not increase your pain. You need to begin a gradual, progressive conditioning program, ideally one that is prescribed just for you and which takes your medical situation into account. This conditioning will include some aerobic component, not only to improve your endurance, but because of its beneficial effect of raising your pain tolerance while helping to discharge the tensions which develop each day from having to cope with pain as well as with routine daily hassles. As part of this conditioning you will also need to stop using stimulants such as caffeine and nicotine because they contribute to muscle irritability and tightness and thus make pain worse.

6. *Learn how to relax, and practice relaxation regularly.*

Use whatever relaxation technique works best for you, and get really good at it. Then you will be able to avoid muscle tension, which makes pain worse and tends to tire you quickly. When you take breaks to pace yourself, these relaxation techniques can be very refreshing and helpful in restoring your energy level. With some of them, such as self-hypnosis and imagery, you can block out pain and learn to split your awareness in such a way that you don't feel the pain, although it is still there—somewhere. As with the physical-conditioning exercises, you will have to practice relaxation daily in order to maintain your proficiency and get the benefits.

7. *Keep yourself busy.*

The reason for having specific goals for work or worklike activities, recreation or hobbies and social activities is not just to bring you satisfaction, although that is very important. It is also to have plenty to do. You need to keep busy so as to be involved in what you are doing and not in your pain. When you are absorbed in these activities, you are not dwelling on the pain, and it cannot bother you as much. You are keeping your attention focused on things outside of yourself, and so are not noticing the pain. Whenever the pain (or feeling discouraged) seems to start getting the upper hand, immediately change what you are doing and thinking about. "Move your muscles, change your thoughts," and switch from one activity to another.

8. *Pace your activities.*

Learn what your time limits are for each activity, and stop before the pain increases. Take relaxation breaks, listening to your tapes and letting yourself relax completely at least twice daily. At other times, switch from one activity to another so that different muscles and different kinds of mental activities are involved. At still other times, you may repeat certain of your exercises, such as back exercises. The principle here is that remaining in one position or repeating one particular activity too long can result in increased awareness of pain. Following a schedule to change activities regularly will allow you to pace yourself better, and you will be able to accomplish a lot and be absorbed in what you are doing and yet not have any worsening of the pain.

9. *Have your family and friends support only your healthy behavior, not your invalidism.*

You need to talk to them about not asking about your pain or offering to do things for you that you can do for yourself. You should not use your pain as a way of bullying others, making them feel guilty or getting out of things that you should be doing. You need to have family and friends give you emotional support and pats on the back for acting normal, not for being disabled and in pain. When people fuss over you for being in pain, it keeps you involved in your pain and disability, and both seem worse than they need to. It is more satisfying and a better distraction from the pain to have the attention and praise for all you're accomplishing despite the pain.

10. *Be open and reasonable with your doctor.*

Your doctor would be very pleased to be able to eliminate your pain if that were possible, but if it were possible, then you wouldn't have chronic pain. Don't insist on relief when none is to be had, nor on prescriptions for narcotics, which will only make the problem worse in the long run. What you should expect is a periodic reevaluation of the pain problem to make sure nothing is being overlooked and that the pain is not part of a progressive disease. And you can expect to be kept up to date on new developments in pain treatments that might help you. Remember that chronic pain is not an emergency and pain flare-ups can be kept to a minimum better by your following the principles in this book than by your frantic phone calls to the doctor.

11. *Practice effective empathy with others having pain problems.*
Misery loves company, if that company knows what it's like to be miserable. You should join with other pain patients for sharing techniques for overcoming pain (*not* to talk about the pain) and for emotional support.

Groups of patients, such as those in the American Chronic Pain Association, can lobby for more governmental support of pain research and can support private organizations, like the International Pain Foundation, which are engaged in research and educational activities. And your group may wish to support organizations like Amnesty International in their campaign to end the practice of torture, because chronic-pain patients can appreciate as no other group can what torture victims are suffering (see Appendix B). Through these political activities you can feel as though you are making a useful contribution in an area—pain—in which you are an expert. There is satisfaction in striking a blow against pain wherever in the world it is. In that satisfaction you will receive at least as much as you give.

12. *Remain hopeful.*
From time to time you may feel worn out and discouraged, and this is to be expected. But the feeling will pass, especially as you change your activities and your thoughts. It also helps to remember the wide range of ongoing pain research, which

will undoubtedly continue to yield new understanding and breakthroughs. There have been many great advances in just the past fifteen years, and some pain conditions which had previously been untreatable are now routinely treated with great success. There is every reason to hope that more and more answers and new techniques will be forthcoming. There is every reason to remain optimistic.

Appendix A:
Some Pain Centers in the United States

Most people will be able to read the ideas in this book and, with the advice and supervision of their doctors, work out a program for themselves for living better despite the pain. But others, because of different kinds of pain problems and different kinds of personal difficulties, may need the organization and direction of a pain management program.

Finding a good pain center that is best for you is difficult. The best source of information is your own doctor. He or she may have sent other patients to a local pain center, or heard good things from colleagues or patients about a local program. That is usually the best kind of referral.

For those who do not have a good nearby program or center, the following list of pain centers is offered. This is by no means a complete list. Many excellent centers may be omitted, and the fact that any pain clinic or center or treatment program is not listed here should not be considered in any way a judgment about it—what follows is only a partial listing of some four dozen pain centers which have established programs meeting minimum standards of staffing and record keeping and evaluation and treatment. If you do not find a nearby pain center on this list, and your doctor does not know of one, you might try calling the medical school or university hospital nearest you—many of them have fine pain management programs or know of good ones in your vicinity.

I must add that attending one of these programs, like reading this book, is not an automatic guarantee that you will attain pain relief. Obviously, there can be no such guarantee. You can get from the program only what you put into it, and even at best most people are going to continue to have some pain. These programs, and the techniques you learn and practice, can only help you to cope better, but that is something after all, and it may make a great difference.

Spain Rehabilitation Center
1717 Sixth Avenue South
Birmingham, AL 35233
(205) 934-4011

The Center
Mesa Lutheran Hospital
525 West Brown Road
Mesa, AZ 85201
(602) 834-1211

St. Joseph's Hospital and Medical
    Center
350 West Thomas Road
Phoenix, AZ 85013
(602) 285-3474

St. Jude Hospital and
    Rehabilitation Center
101 East Valencia Mesa Drive
Fullerton, CA 92632
(714) 871-3280

Rehabilitation Institute
Glendale Adventist Medical Center
1509 Wilson Terrace
Glendale, CA 91206
(213) 240-8000

Center for Diagnostic and
    Rehabilitation Medicine
Daniel Freeman Hospital Medical
    Center
333 North Prairie Avenue
Inglewood, CA 90301
(213) 674-7050

New Directions Rehabilitation
    Center
Centinela Hospital Medical Center
Post Office Box 720
Inglewood, CA 90307
(213) 673-4660

Pain Treatment Center
Scripps Clinic & Research
  Foundation
10666 North Torrey Pines Road
La Jolla, CA 92037
(619) 455-8898

Pain Center
Scripps Memorial Hospital
Post Office Box 28
La Jolla, CA 92038
(619) 457-6952

Center for Rehabilitation Medicine
Northridge Hospital Medical
  Center
18300 Roscoe Boulevard
Morthridge, CA 91328
(213) 885-8500

New Hope Pain Center
55 East California Boulevard
Pasadena, CA 91105-3202
(818) 405-8000

Casa Colina Hospital for
  Rehabilitative Medicine
255 East Bonita Avenue
Pomona, CA 91767
(714) 593-7521

Center for Rehabilitation Medicine
Valley Hospital Medical Center
14500 Sherman Circle
Van Nuys, CA 91405
(818) 908-8676

Boulder Pain Control Center
4850 Sterling Drive
Boulder, CO 80301
(303) 444-7400

Rehabilitation Center
Boulder Memorial Hospital
311 Mapleton Avenue
Boulder, CO 80302
(303) 443-0230

Spalding Rehabilitation Hospital
1919 Ogden Street
Denver, CO 80218
(303) 861-0504

Hilltop Rehabilitation Hospital
1100 Patterson Road
Grand Junction, CO 81505
(303) 244-6007

Pain Management Center
3599 University Boulevard
  South, Suite 1
Jacksonville, FL 32216
(904) 391-1250

Andrew G. Frank Rehabilitation
  Institute
12405 N.E. Sixth Avenue
North Miami, FL 33161
(305) 895-6666

The Pain Management Program at
  Behavioral Health and
  Rehabilitation Associates, Inc.
5330 Diplomat Circle
Orlando, FL 32810
(305) 629-1366

Rehabilitation Institute of West
 Florida
Post Office Box 18900
Pensacola, FL 32523-8900
(904) 474-5358

Center for Rehabilitation Medicine
Emory University Hospital
1441 Clifton Road N.E.
Atlanta, GA 30322
(404) 329-5507

DeKalb Pain Management and
 Rehabilitation
484 Irvin Court, Suite 260
Decatur, GA 30030
(404) 299-1060

Pain Treatment Center
Lake Forest Hospital
660 North Westmoreland Road
Lake Forest, IL 60045
(312) 234-5600

Mercy Pain Center
Mercy Hospital Medical Center
1188 Third Street
Des Moines, IA 50314
(515) 247-4430

Physical Medicine and
 Rehabilitation Center
Physicians & Surgeons Hospital
Post Office Box 4466
Shreveport, LA 71104
(318) 227-3950

Center for Pain Management and
 Orthopedic Surgery
8830 Cameron Street
Silver Spring, MD 20910
(301) 587-2500

Boston Pain Center
A division of Spalding
 Rehabilitation Hospital
125 Nashua Street
Boston, MA 02114
(617) 720-6668

New England Rehabilitation
 Hospital
One Rehabilitation Way
Woburn, MA 01801
(671) 935-5050

Shealy Pain and Health
 Rehabilitation Institute
3525 South National, Suite 207
Springfield, MO 65807
(417) 882-0850

Jean Hanna Clark Rehabilitation
 Center
1001 Shadow Lane
Las Vegas, NV 89106
(702) 385-5212

Betty Bacharach Rehabilitation
 Hospital
Jim Leeds Road
Pomona, NJ 08240
(609) 652-7000

Margaret W. Strong Pain Clinic
Santa Fe Neurological Sciences
  Institute
531 Harkle Road, Suite B
Santa Fe, NM 87501
(505) 983-4744

Orthopaedic-Arthritis Pain Center/
  Hospital for Joint Diseases/
  Orthopaedic Institute
301 East 17th Street
New York, NY 10003
(212) 598-6000

Sunnyview Hospital and
  Rehabilitation Center
1270 Belmont Avenue
Schenectady, NY 12308
(518) 382-4500

Dodd Hall
Ohio State University Hospital
472 West Eighth Avenue
Columbus, OH 43210
(614) 422-5547

The Pain Center
Miami Valley Hospital
1 Wyoming Street
Dayton, OH 45409
(513) 220-2723

Good Samaritan Medical Center
  and Rehabilitation Center
800 Forest Avenue
Zanesville, OH 43701
(614) 454-5469

Emmanuel Rehabilitation Center
3001 North Gantenbein
Portland, OR 97229
(503) 280-4400

Northwest Pain Center
10615 S.E. Cherry Blossom Drive
Portland, OR 97216
(503) 256-1930

Magee Rehabilitation Hospital
6 Franklin Plaza
Philadelphia, PA 19102
(215) 864-7100

Roger C. Peace Rehabilitation
  Hospital
Greenville Hospital Center
701 Grove Road
Greenville, SC 29605
(803) 242-7703

Middle Tennessee Back Care
  Center
209 Ward Circle, Maryland Farms
Brentwood, TN 37027
(615) 377-3088

Baptist Memorial Hospital -
  Regional Rehabilitation Center
1025 E. H. Crump Boulevard
Memphis, TN 38104
(901) 522-6550

Multidisciplinary Pain Center
University of Washington
Seattle, WA 98195
(206) 548-4284

Rehabilitation Department
St. Joseph Hospital and Health
  Care Center
Post Office Box 2197
Tacoma, WA 98405
(206) 627-4101

Curative Rehabilitation Center
9001 Watertown Plank Road
Wauwatosa, WI 53226
(414) 259-1414

Pain Management Unit
Waukesha Memorial Hospital
725 American Avenue
Waukesha, WI 53186
(414) 544-2011

Those who do not feel pain seldom think that it is felt.
—*Samuel Johnson*

There are several items relating to pain which are worth considering separately. They have a bearing on your own pain, some directly, some indirectly. Each involves politics to a degree. There appears to be a strange connection between pain and politics. We have already noted that politics slowed the original acceptance of analgesia and anesthesia into regular use in medicine. The same occurred when hypnosis was demonstrated to control the pain of amputating a leg; some distinguished scientists and doctors said it couldn't have done so, that the patient must have been faking, and others said that people *should* suffer pain during surgery and ordered the demonstration removed from the record. There has not been much improvement in such attitudes, and now we will see some ways in which this is so.

Neglect and Opposition

The Nuprin Pain Report, published in 1985, was the first survey of the frequency and extent of pain in adults in the continental United States. As noted earlier, one of its findings was that 12.8 percent of adult Americans reported having significant pain at least 101 days during the preceding year. In other words, nearly 20.8 million persons have chronic or frequently recurring pain. The numbers would be greater if those under eighteen had been included.

And yet, despite the fact that so many people are afflicted with chronic pain, and that it cost the economy $55 billion in loss of productivity from full-time workers alone, there has been very great neglect of this problem. Notice that a private company, Bristol-Myers, distributors of the nonprescription analgesic Nuprin, had to commission the survey, which was carried out by Louis Harris & Associates, a private survey research firm.

Why was all this done privately, at considerable expense? Because no government agency, including the National Institutes of Health, had ever performed such an obvious study. Yet, before you try to work on any problem it is obviously important to know something about its extent. Federal funding of research in pain has been very inadequate, and so there is a great deal that is still unknown about some very basic questions. (As this is written in 1986 I have just received notice that the National Center for Health Statistics is preparing proposals for a more thorough and extensive survey of chronic pain in the United States.)

Why has there been this lag in pain research? It is probably because we are used to thinking of advances in health research in terms of traditional diseases. The country has many private organizations and foundations drumming up popular support for certain diseases, such as the Arthritis Foundation, the

American Cancer Society, The American Heart Association, Shriners Burn Institutes, etc. And although pain is usually a serious part of such diseases, these organizations don't do their fund raising around the issue of pain and its control, but rather they stress the need to find cures.

In the same way, the National Institute of Health is organized around the traditional diseases, such as the National Institute on Arthritis and Related Diseases, the National Cancer Institute, etc. And in each of these institutes, only a very small percentage of the budget is given to research on the nature of pain in that disease and ways of preventing or controlling it. And one of the reasons that organizations are built around traditional diseases is that the medical specialties developed that way, with medical scientists receiving their training in specialties like arthritis (rheumatology), cancer (oncology), etc., and teaching and doing research in medical school departments and hospitals, which are similarly organized. It is just part of the history of medicine that researchers didn't specialize in symptoms like nausea, fever or pain, which were associated with many diseases, but rather in the diseases, which were associated with many symptoms.

It is also true that researchers go where research grant money is, and in this country the money is where the medical lobbyists raise it. Cancer, heart disease and arthritis are "sexy" causes—and currently the autoimmune deficiency syndrome (AIDS) is, as well—and money is raised for basic research to find cures. There is virtually no interest in allocating funds for pain as a symptom of such diseases—although it is a significant symptom indeed.

In addition to such historical neglect, there has actually been active opposition to finding alternatives to narcotics for pain control. While the federal government has been pushing its war on illegal use and transportation of narcotics—and spending many millions on this which could be spent on research on pain control—there has been a continuing effort on the part of pharmaceutical firms to come up with new and more effective analgesics that do not have the drawbacks of the present ones.

The marketing divisions of these firms spend heavily to advertise in medical journals, hoping thereby to influence physicians to prescribe their products. The effect of all this is to reinforce in doctors the impulse to think of prescription analgesics as the way of controlling pain. As a result, safe and effective alternatives to these substances are under-researched and under-used.

In fact, one large drug company in recent years bought up a successful TENS company, then suppressed its sales so that the sales of analgesics wouldn't be hurt. (The management of the TENS division sued the parent company on that charge, and won!) So it is obvious that not only research, but drug sales, and the education of physicians and public are all influenced by where the money is.

Recent Trends

There has been a very recent development which has started to have an effect on the indifference and opposition to research on pain. This has come about through the development of pain treatment centers in this country and elsewhere. These centers (clinics, programs) were started initially by those who had been doing pain research in their different specialties (anesthesiology, neurosurgery, psychology, etc.) and who realized that only by forming specialized pain clinics would they be able to combine their expertise to come up with treatments that would provide patients with the best of available knowledge and skills.

From these beginnings, the different specialists were able

both to stimulate research into new areas and develop applications of such alternative techniques as behavioral and cognitive training, neurostimulation, biofeedback, etc. Various pain centers began to publish the results of their treatment programs, and as these successes were greater than had ever been seen before in the managing of chronic pain, more and more attention has been given to the problem both by the medical community and by the public. As a consequence, there has been more pressure put on the National Institutes of Health and the private foundations to fund research on pain.

There is increasing funding now for basic research on the nature of pain and on the mechanisms of analgesia, chemical and otherwise. There is new interest in pain measurement (we don't even have a "pain thermometer"!). There is a growing interest in evaluating the data from the pain clinics to see what are the most effective techniques for controlling different kinds of pain. And there is even discussion now about better ways of informing physicians and the public about alternative methods for pain control. All of these developments are still quite new, but they are a beginning.

As part of this trend, some patients and their families and friends have started to organize as well. This is very important, because our advances in being able to understand and control pain will depend to a large extent on how effectively these groups can organize and lobby and exert political influence.

One group of professionals—researchers, doctors and nurses—formed the International Association for the Study of Pain to promote research and to publish the results in the journal. *Pain.* They have created a foundation to raise funds in support of such research and to educate both professionals and the public in new techniques of pain control. Those who would like to help with this should contact:

International Pain Foundation
909 N.E. 43rd Street
Seattle, WA 98105
(206) 547-2157
Marie Leonard, Executive
Officer

Chronic-pain patients, some of whom have been treated in various pain treatment centers, have begun an organization called The American Chronic Pain Association. This is a self-help support organization for individuals with chronic pain. It supplies information and suggestions, and is forming chapters in different areas where patients will be able to give each other more direct support. Such organizations have the possibility of lobbying legislators and foundations so that more research and better treatment of pain can become available. You can find out more about this from:

The American Chronic Pain Association
257 Old Haymaker Road
Monroeville, PA 15146
(412) 856-9676
Penny Cowan, Executive
Director

The Fellowship of Pain

The Fellowship of those who bear the Mark of Pain. Who are the members of this Fellowship? Those who have learnt by experience what physical pain and bodily anguish mean, belong together all the world over; they are united by a secret bond.

—Albert Schweitzer

Those who work with people in pain see a great deal of suffering and anguish every day. We see the effects of disease and injury and age, and all that these things do to individuals and their friends and families. When we think as well of the human misery from other natural causes, such as hunger and malnutrition, disasters due to earthquakes and floods and fires, etc., it seems as though humankind has more than enough unhappiness to go around.

Therefore it is a shock to learn of humans deliberately inflicting pain on one another, not just occasionally in a moment of anger, but coldly, cruelly, systematically, on a widespread scale. We find it hard to understand, and the scope of it difficult to comprehend. But in scores of countries around the world, thousands and thousands of people are tortured. Not in the past, not yesterday, but today. Right now, as you are reading this, there are men and women and children writhing in pain and screaming in agony as the most fiendish things imaginable are done to them.

How do we know this? There have been careful investigations and documentation by reputable individuals and organizations, who have interviewed victims and, in some instances, those who have carried out the torture as well. Stories have been double-checked, verified by others and supported by the evidence on the tortured bodies. There have been photographs, eyewitness reports, records kept by jailers, etc.

These horrifying events are known to be happening right now on a large scale in countries dominated by either right-wing or left-wing dictatorships in every part of the world. The torture is used to terrify the people, since it is inflicted not just on members of the opposition but on ordinary working people.

Two books have recently been published which document and describe what is happening, and they are a terrible indictment of the capacity of people to be cruel to one another. They are a record of torture, which seems to be escalating and becoming ever more widespread. These books are:

- Amnesty International. *Torture in the Eighties.* Amnesty International Publications, London, 1984.
- Eric Stover and Elena O. Nightingale, M.D., Editors (for the American Association for the Advancement of Science): *The Breaking of Bodies and Minds: Torture, Psychiatric Abuse, and the Health Professions.* W. H. Freeman, New York, 1985.

Each of these books describes, in a different way, where and how and why torture is being performed, and on whom, and what the effects are. They also list organizations that are giving help and hope to the victims, and attempts to bring about an end to such awful acts. You can probably find these books at your local library, or order them through a bookstore.

If you have chronic pain, or know someone who does, you understand very well what the victims of torture are feeling and the effects long-continued pain has on them. You can feel a special kind of sympathy for them. And remember, they are not given any analgesics nor any opportunities for other forms of pain relief. Everything possible is done to make the pain worse, not better. If you, yourself, are being tortured by the effects of pain due to some injury or disease, you have the possibility of getting help to control or reduce your pain. They have no hope, unless others work to help them.

I believe that those who have pain, together with those professionals who do pain research and treat pain patients, belong to a special Fellowship, as Dr. Schweitzer said. We have a special empathy for and understanding of those who suffer pain. And I believe that we, more than any others, have a special obligation to do whatever we can to help torture victims, because of being united by this bond. As we would want others to help us with our suffering, if they could, so we must help other pain victims, if we can.

Those who want to learn more should write to:

Amnesty International USA
304 West 58th Street
New York, NY 10019

As Dr. Schweitzer wrote: "Those who have learnt by experience what physical pain and bodily anguish mean, belong together all the world over."

Index